1983

Test-Tube

Test-Tube Babies

Test-Tube Babies

A guide to moral questions,
present techniques and future
possibilities

Edited by
William A. W. Walters and
Peter Singer

Melbourne
Oxford University Press
Oxford Auckland New York

OXFORD UNIVERSITY PRESS
Oxford London Glasgow New York Toronto
Delhi Bombay Calcutta Madras Karachi
Kuala Lumpur Singapore Hong Kong Tokyo
Nairobi Dar es Salaam Cape Town
Melbourne Auckland

and associate companies in

Beirut Berlin Ibadan Mexico City Nicosia

National Library of Australia
Cataloguing-in-Publication data:

Walters, William A. W. and Singer, Peter
Test-Tube Babies
ISBN 0 19 554342 4 (case)
ISBN 0 19 554340 8 (paperback)
1. Fertilization in vitro, Human — Moral
and religious aspects. 2. Human embryo —
Transplantation — Moral and religious aspects.
Singer, Peter, 1946-. II. Walters, William A. W.
(Series: Series 500).
174'.2

Typeset in Melbourne by Meredith Typesetters
Printed in Melbourne by Globe Press Pty. Ltd.
Published by Oxford University Press, 7 Bowen Crescent, Melbourne

CONTENTS

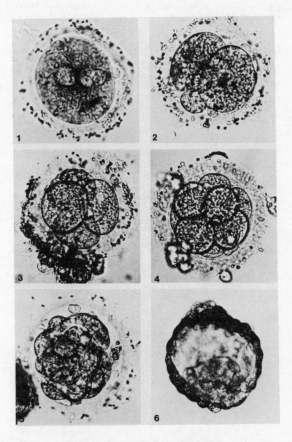

Preimplantation Human Embryos

Photograph key: 1.* A 1-cell human embryo 12 hours after fertilization; 2.* A 2-cell human embryo 30 hours; 3.* A 4-cell human embryo 40 hours; 4.* An 8-cell human embryo 55 hours; 5. A morula stage human embryo 100 hours; 6. A blastocyst stage human embryo 140 hours after fertilization.

* indicates stage at which embryos are transferred back into the uterus.

All these embryos have been photographed alive, in sterile culture media, using a non-invasive technique.

(Reproduced with permission from The Journal of Reproduction and Fertility, and the authors, Trounson, A.O., Mohr, L., Wood, C. and Leeton, J.F.)

Preface

In many respects this book is a result of the pioneering in vitro fertilization (IVF) and embryo transfer (ET) work of Professor Carl Wood and his group at Monash University, the Queen Victoria Medical Centre, and St Andrew's Hospital, Melbourne.

From the very beginning of the work, which was aimed at relieving infertility in married couples, the Queen Victoria Medical Centre Ethics Committee started discussions about the associated ethical problems. In addition, several special meetings, to which a number of ethicists in Melbourne were asked to contribute, were held. More recently, members of the newly established Human Bioethics Centre at Monash University have also contributed to these discussions.

Because of the current public interest and concern about IVF, we thought that it would be profitable to gather together the different points of view on the ethical aspects of IVF expressed at the various meetings we have had on the subject — hence this book.

We wish to emphasize that the authors of chapters have expressed their own views: their contributions do not necessarily mean that they are in agreement with views expressed elsewhere in the book. Likewise we, as editors, in those chapters we have written, cannot claim to represent the opinions of the other authors. Furthermore, although various points of view have been presented, this book does not in any way claim to be entirely comprehensive of ethical aspects of IVF.

We would like to thank Christine Simpson and Jean Archer for their help in typing and other tasks related to the preparation of the manuscript; and we are also grateful to James Hall of Oxford University Press for his advice and encouragement.

William A. W. Walters
Department of Obstetrics and Gynaecology
Monash University

Peter Singer
Department of Philosophy
Monash University

1 IVF and ET: What it is and how it works

John F. Leeton, Alan O. Trounson, and *Carl Wood*

Human fertility depends upon the successful fertilization of a human egg in the outer end of the Fallopian tube, its subsequent transport from the tube into the uterus after about three days, and its implantation there. In about 30 per cent of women, a pregnancy with the delivery of a live baby can be expected.[1] The functions of the Fallopian tubes, therefore, include the collection of the egg when it is discharged from the ovary at about the middle of the menstrual cycle, transportation of the sperm from the uterus to the outer end of the tube where the sperm meet the egg and fertilization occurs, and nutrition and transport of the resulting early developing embryo down the tube to the uterine cavity.

The original reason for attempting in vitro fertilization (IVF), which means the exposure of the egg to sperm outside of the body in laboratory glassware, was to by-pass damaged or blocked tubes where their function was inadequate to produce a normal pregnancy. Originally the aim of IVF was to replace tubal function by bringing the sperm into contact with the egg *in vitro* and then to transfer the embryo into the uterus (ET). Implantation and pregnancy resulting from this technique is identical with that of a pregnancy conceived by sexual intercourse.

Indications for IVF

One of the most common reasons for attempting IVF and ET is unsuccessful tubal surgery. More than one of these operations may have been performed and the treatment may have been by ordinary surgical techniques or by those using high power magnification with an operating microscope. The overall success rate of tubal surgery is only about 30 per cent,[2] and the development of micro-surgical techniques has only improved these results by about 10 per cent.[3]

Tubal surgery may be considered impossible in those cases with extensive tubal disease where the resulting tubal function would remain poor. Tubal pregnancy is a serious complication of tubal surgery, and some women will therefore not accept a major surgical reconstructive procedure, although they still wish to resolve their problem of tubal infertility.

Infertility of unknown cause occurs in about 10 per cent of infertility cases and has a poor outlook for achieving pregnancy when its duration is over four years. Many investigations and empirical treatments are usually attempted in these cases often at great expense and emotional distress. Treatments include surgery, for example, suspension of the uterus, artificial insemination by either husband's semen (AIH) or semen donated by another man (AID), or both, and various forms of drug therapy to attempt to improve either egg or sperm production. It is possible that there are undetected abnormalities in the eggs or sperm, or factors which inhibit fertilization. IVF may therefore be used as a diagnostic test to determine whether abnormalities of the egg or sperm cells or their transport are causing infertility. This concept will be discussed later in the chapter.

Another group of women with infertility which may be considered suitable for IVF is that comprising women who, although having no problems after routine infertility tests, fail to conceive after more than one year with AID treatment.

Finally, IVF and ET are being explored in the treatment of male infertility where the number, movement or structure of the sperm are considered to be abnormal. Successful fertilization has been obtained in the case of men with concentrations of sperm as low as 5 million per millilitre of semen, the normal count ranging from 20 to 100 million sperm per millilitre of semen. When sperm numbers are markedly reduced, however, there is often a high incidence of sperm abnormalities which may impair the effectiveness of IVF. Furthermore, no pregnancies have been obtained when the sperm movements are less than 40 per cent of those seen normally. Frozen semen containing sperm with movements greater than 40 per cent of those seen normally can be successfully used for IVF.

Selection Procedures

Reproductive efficiency declines with increasing age and the successful outcome of IVF and ET is also thought to follow this trend. Women over the age of thirty-five are excluded in some centres, although the Monash University programme accepts women up to the age of forty-five.

Previous childbearing suggests that factors contributing to infertility, with the exception of tubal disease, are unlikely to be present. Women who have already had a child also have a significantly better chance of an easy ET because the neck of the womb, having been stretched during delivery of a baby, is wider. In some centres women with more than one child are excluded from the IVF programme, although this is not the policy of the Monash University team.

Religious beliefs may prevent a couple accepting IVF and ET. After an explanation of the procedures, the final decision is made by the couple.

The couple must be able to cope, both physically and emotionally, with IVF and ET, pregnancy, birth, and the subsequent rearing of the child. Most infertile couples have emotional problems related to their infertility, and unsuccessful treatments often increase their anxiety. In some situations psychological counselling may be beneficial. Our infertile couples undergoing IVF have formed a support group called the 'IVF Friends', one of whose objectives is mutual assistance with the emotional problems associated with infertility, both by self-help and group discussion.

Egg production and maturity must be confirmed by biochemical testing, and an examination of ejaculated seminal fluid should be within acceptable limits. At least two analyses of seminal fluid are carried out before IVF treatment commences.

Laparoscopy entails the passage of a telescope into the abdominal cavity through a very small incision in the abdominal wall. It allows inspection of the internal organs and collection of eggs from the ovaries. The procedure is done under general anaesthesia. It is mandatory for all women undergoing IVF to have relatively accessible ovaries for egg collection, which is determined by a preliminary laparoscopy.

Preparation for IVF

Couples should be informed in detail of all aspects of IVF and ET before entry into the programme. This is usually done by at least one extensive consultation with the husband, wife, and gynaecologist, as well as an appointment at the special IVF clinic where various members of the medical team are present for consultation. A member of the patients' support group, who has experienced the IVF procedure, is also available for advice and to help with arrangements. Informal lectures by members of the IVF team, group discussions, and the showing of videotapes describing the IVF procedure are held regularly. Instruction brochures and booklets about the procedures are also provided.

Husband and wife sign a consent form which includes a statement that the risks of the procedures have been explained, that success is not guaranteed, that the possibility of foetal malformation exists, and that foetal diagnostic tests which aim to detect foetal malformation are available.

The Clinical Procedures

Timing of egg collection is critical and aims to obtain a mature egg from one of the ovaries immediately before its expulsion from the ovary. If this timing is premature, the egg is not fully mature and cannot be fertilized normally. On the other hand, if the egg has already been expelled from the ovary it may not be found. It was originally thought that normal spontaneous egg-producing cycles were necessary for successful IVF and ET, but the Monash team has shown that egg production can be stimulated with fertility drugs thereby allowing better results from IVF than those achieved in the normal non-stimulated cycle.[4]

Stimulation of egg production increases the chance of obtaining one or more eggs. Furthermore, if two or more eggs become fertilized and develop into embryos, the chance of establishing pregnancy is substantially increased by the transfer of two embryos back into the uterus instead of one.[5] The basic aim of the transfer of two embryos is to improve the overall pregnancy rate, while accepting that a proportion of such pregnancies will result in twins.

Stimulated egg production also has advantages in the organization of IVF because the time of egg maturation in the ovary can be predicted with greater accuracy. The length of the woman's stay in hospital before laparoscopy is thereby reduced, and the timing of the operation can be better planned. Stimulation of egg production is achieved by prescribing clomiphene citrate tablets (fertility pills) or human pituitary gonadotrophins (fertility injections) in varying dose schedules.

Egg development is as important as the timing of surgery in relation to egg pick-up. The ovaries must be clearly accessible for the collection of mature eggs, and a satisfactory collecting system must be used.

The ovary is held by forceps that have been introduced into the abdominal cavity adjacent to the laparoscope so that one or more of its egg follicles can be gently punctured and aspirated under vision by a special 23 cm long needle which is inserted between the laparoscope and the forceps. This needle is lined by teflon tubing which is continuous with the collecting test-tube, so that the flow of follicular fluid is constant, and turbulence is reduced.[6] This needle and collecting system allows an egg collection rate of 90 per cent and reduces the risk of damage to the egg in its passage from the ovary to the collecting tube.

IVF and Embryo Culture

Methods of IVF and embryo culture are highly specialized and have evolved from exhaustive physiological studies carried out in laboratory and domestic animals. Experience, skill, and strict quality control of all laboratory procedures are needed for successful IVF. Human eggs and embryos are too valuable to use in establishing the suitability of culture media or procedures. Therefore mouse embryos have been used for quality control assays and as models for testing the validity of new procedures introduced into the IVF programme.[7]

A fresh semen sample obtained by masturbation is provided in the hospital ninety minutes before insemination of the eggs. The sperm is washed and centrifuged twice with culture medium resulting in a final concentration of 100 000 to 800 000 motile sperm in the final tube for insemination.

The eggs are cultured in the laboratory for five to six hours to allow them to complete their maturation process before they are inseminated. This time lag has a physiological basis as the eggs have been collected before they are fully ripe: the delay has produced a higher proportion of embryos.

Fertilization of an egg can be clearly seen microscopically twelve to twenty-three hours after insemination and is detected by the presence of two pronuclei, one from the sperm and one from the egg. A range of culture media has been used successfully and a single culture medium can be used for both fertilization and embryo culture. After approximately thirty hours the fertilized egg may divide into a two-cell embryo which in about forty hours may divide into a four-cell embryo and at approximately sixty hours into an eight-cell embryo.

ET

Pregnancies have developed following the transfer of one-cell to sixteen-cell human embryos. Older embryos are not used because they do not develop beyond sixteen cells in the Fallopian tube under normal circumstances. Prolonged culture is thought to promote degeneration of the embryo. Currently the Monash team is transferring embryos at the one- to eight-cell stage, although the optimum stage of embryo development for transfer in the human has not yet been established.

The normal embryo is transferred into the uterine cavity by a narrow transparent teflon catheter passed through the neck of the uterus. This route has the advantage of being simple, safe, painless, and requiring no anaesthesia. The husband is encouraged to be present with his wife during the ET procedure. The embryo is placed in a minute volume of culture fluid in the catheter which is then passed slowly and gently through the neck of the uterus to the top of the uterine cavity. The fluid containing the embryo is gently injected into the uterus from the catheter by a syringe after which the catheter is slowly withdrawn. Any slight bleeding or pain during this critical procedure will compromise the future development of the embryo. Pregnancies in the Monash programme have only resulted following relatively easy passage of the catheter.

The woman rests in hospital for twenty-four hours and afterwards at home she limits her activities for several days, but no special precautions are taken or restrictions advised. Weekly blood hormone levels are measured for the first twelve weeks after ET to diagnose pregnancy and its early development.

Success Rate of IVF

Success rates may be reported in several ways. Expressing the success rate per laparoscopy has the advantage of taking into account the physical risk, serious inconvenience, and most of the cost to each patient. The results of the Monash team during June-December 1980 from 112 laparoscopies were twelve clinical pregnancies. Seven were in patients with tubal damage, four were in those with unexplained infertility, and one resulted from the transfer of an embryo fertilized by donor sperm as the husband's sperm failed to fertilize the wife's eggs. Three of these pregnancies miscarried and the remaining nine pregnancies produced ten babies, one set of twins being included. These success rates are now comparable with those following some surgical procedures for treating infertility caused by tubal damage.

Current Uses of IVF and ET

The most common reason for using IVF and ET is to attempt to overcome tubal infertility as a result of either diseased or blocked Fallopian tubes. A small but significant success rate can now be achieved in this situation. IVF and ET can also be tried in the treatment of endometriosis which is a chronic disease of the ovaries that is associated with infertility. The Monash team has achieved one pregnancy in a woman with this long-standing problem. The technique of IVF and ET has also produced pregnancies in women with unexplained infertility. The success rate of treating unexplained infertility by IVF is comparable to that obtained for treating infertility as a result of tubal disorders. As the IVF and ET procedures are optimized these success rates will improve.

IVF is a new technique which may be used for diagnostic as well as therapeutic purposes. In women with unexplained infertility, IVF can be used to diagnose the level of the fertility defect, that is, abnormalities in sperm, eggs, fertilization, or tubal transport. Because normal IVF and embryo growth rates are less than 50 per cent, a control system is needed when testing the sperm-egg interaction in unexplained infertility. This control is applied by placing one egg with fertile matched donor sperm as well as another similar egg with the husband's sperm.

Successful fertilization with the husband's sperm followed by pregnancy after ET would indicate that some immunological, chemical or physical barrier is preventing pregnancy. Failure to initiate pregnancy following ET may indicate abnormal uterine function which prevents embryo implantation. Fertilization with donor sperm but not with husband's sperm indicates sperm abnormalities in the latter. Finally, in cases where eggs cannot be fertilized by either the husband's or donor sperm, abnormalities of the egg may be responsible.

In those situations where only a donor-matched inseminated embryo is cultured, the couple has to decide whether to accept this embryo or not. This situation has already resulted in a successful pregnancy.[8] If pregnancy does not result, the couple is advised to proceed with artificial insemination by donor sperm (AID). In cases where embryos are produced by both husband and donor sperm, the couple has the choice of accepting both embryos. The success rate of pregnancy is significantly improved with two embryos. The couple may refuse to accept the donor-inseminated embryo which, with their consent, could be preserved and stored by deep-freezing for future transfer into another recipient. Embryo freezing is now being investigated.

Embryo Storage
Some women are unsuitable for ET following IVF because of uterine bleeding, general illness, fever, or the inability to pass a catheter through the neck of the womb at ET. A method for embryo storage by freezing would allow time to correct these problems so that transfer could be carried out during a later egg-producing cycle. In addition, the collection of several eggs may develop after IVF into two or more embryos. Those embryos which are additional to the number requested by the woman for transfer during that treatment cycle could be freeze-stored for thawing and transfer in a later egg-producing cycle. The alternatives that would need consideration if freeze-storing techniques were not available are either disposal or use for further research interests, for example, embryo structure or biochemistry. These alternatives are considered less desirable than the freezing techniques.

Donor embryos for infertile recipients may be indicated when IVF is impossible in an infertile woman because her ovaries are either absent, diseased, or hidden by pelvic adhesions that prevent their visualization at laparoscopy. The sperm of the infertile woman's husband could be used for IVF of the donor's egg. This biological situation is parallel to AID and needs the same careful ethical and legal considerations. To achieve ET from a donor to a recipient, it would be necessary to either synchronize the egg-producing cycles of the donor and the recipient using hormone therapy or freeze the donor embryo for subsequent thawing and transfer to the recipient at the correct stage of her egg-producing cycle.

So far no pregnancy has developed following the transfer of a freeze-thawed human embryo, although it has been shown that human embryos beyond the eight-cell stage of development may survive freezing and thawing and continue to develop in culture.

In our clinic women are advised that the survival rate of embryos following freeze-thawing may be very low, but so far all patients have chosen to have their embryos frozen when the appropriate situation has arisen. They are also advised that, from experiences of large numbers of young born after freeze-preservation of animal embryos, foetal abnormality rates for frozen embryos appear to be the same as those for non-frozen embryos and that inbred strains of mice breed true to their genetic constitutions following freezing.[9]

Summary

IVF may be successfully used for both diagnostic and therapeutic purposes. The current success rates for the four basic steps in IVF in our group have been summarized as follows: the rate of egg collection 85 to 90 per cent, the rate of fertilization 80 to 90 per cent, the rate of embryo development 80 to 90 per cent, and the pregnancy rate per laparoscopy 12 to 20 per cent. The success rate of treating unexplained infertility by IVF is comparable to that obtained for treating infertility as a result of tubal disease.

The factors determining a successful outcome are unknown and require much more study. As ET may be difficult in some situations, with IVF being either impossible or unsuccessful, it would seem desirable to attempt successful storage of human embryos by deep-freeze techniques.

2 The Brennan Story:
A small miracle of creation

Peter Roberts

Pippin Jaimee Brennan, the world's thirteenth test-tube baby, was born at 8.13 on Thursday night, a healthy 3.2 kilograms. This is the story of her life from the very beginning.

By 6 p.m., darkness was closing on St Andrew's Hospital in East Melbourne. From the south, squalls threatened rain, sending pedestrians scurrying to the hospital's double doors from cars parked in the deserted streets. Inside, all was quiet. Patients had been fed; visitors were gone. The corridors echoed only hushed voices and the pad-pad of feet.

In a ward on the first floor a group of women in street clothes were sitting on the beds, talking nervously. One of the group had just been wheeled away to an operating theatre nearby as part of Monash University's test-tube baby programme.

Operating theatres hold a fascination for many, a horror for some. At St Andrew's that night a sign written in coloured pen and taped to a glass door said: 'Doctors, this way.' Sterile coats and boots go on over street clothes and you walk inside to a surprise.

Is this an operating theatre? No masses of modern machinery; only a huddle of sterile green figures gathered round a pool of light cast by two overhead lamps. The figures stand hunched over, isolated in a sea of grey-green tiles covering floors and walls. At one end of the operating table is anaesthetist Colin Stewart. His eyes lift only momentarily from a group of dials; his left hand rhythmically pumps a small rubber bag remarkably like a football bladder; his right hand feels the patient's neck for pulse.

Thirty-six hours before, the patient had received the last dose in a course of hormone drugs designed to improve the chances for success in the operation to collect the woman's ova, or eggs. Patients first take clomiphene citrate to stimulate the growth of egg-containing follicles on the ovaries — the body reacts abnormally, producing two, three, four or more eggs. The final injection of human chorionic gonadotrophin precisely times their ripening.

Now the woman lies immobile save for a slowly heaving chest, head turned to one side, eyes taped closed, and mouth filled with tubes carrying the anaesthetist's gases to her lungs. Surgeon John Leeton and his assistant Nick Lolatgis bend over a 20 centimetre square of flesh exposed among the folds of green.

In only a few minutes he has made three small incisions in the abdomen and inserted three instruments. Just below the navel is the laparascope, a combination eyepiece and light that allows the surgeon to look inside the human body. Next in line is a hollow needle only 1 millimetre in diameter and lined with slippery teflon to prevent the egg from sticking. Immediately below are the holding forceps which will search for the ovaries and hold them still. Leeton, a professor of obstetrics at Monash, uses a foot pedal to pump carbon dioxide gas into the woman's abdomen, blowing up the belly for easy access.

Balancing the laparascope against his cheek bones, Leeton hunches over the woman, searching for the left ovary. Using the forceps, he slips back the fimbria, a glove-like membrane that normally contains the ovary and directs expelled eggs into the woman's Fallopian tubes. In this case the tubes are unable to carry out their normal task of transferring eggs to the uterus, and the woman could not normally conceive.

'Here, you have a look,' Leeton says.

The inner body is surprisingly pink, with a darker red ovary clasped firmly by a harsh, inhuman looking metal clamp. Growing on the surface is what looks like a small white button mushroom, lightly criss-crossed with veins; the follicle. Each follicle grows cyst-like on the ovary only to burst and expel its egg on roughly the fourteenth day of the menstrual cycle. The surgeon waits until each follicle is fully ripe. The art lies in piercing the follicle with the hollow needle while at the same time using a foot-operated vacuum pump to gently suck out the egg.

Nick Lolatgis holds a row of small test tubes between thumb and forefinger. A teflon tube starts to flow with a thin honey-coloured liquid drawn from the woman's body. The first tube is filled and removed, and the filing tube is shuffled to the next in line. Anaesthetist Stewart leans over and whispers: 'That is the fluid from the follicle. Hopefully there is going to be an egg in there.'

The hush is shattered as Sister Jillian Wood loudly raps a button on a wall-mounted intercom and says: 'It is coming out.' She wraps her hand around the teflon tube to keep it warm and rushes from the theatre to a nearby laboratory. Several tubes go the same way, leaving the follicle a collapsed sack, pierced by the needle.

The intercom breaks in harshly as Leeton moves to a second follicle: 'We have an egg from tube two.' Two more eggs are announced but still the intercom demands more. The more eggs collected, the greater the chance of fertilization, and the greater the chance of re-implanting a healthy-looking cluster of four or eight cells that have the potential to become a human being.

'Trounson is never satisfied,' says John Leeton.

Across a hallway, on the other end of the intercom, is Dr Alan Trounson, the senior reproductive biologist who handles the eggs through their laboratory fertilization and implantation. A scientist, his background in animal embryology is seen as a key to the success of the Monash team. He looks tired. On one recent weekend he spent all but seven hours at the Queen Victoria Medical Centre or St Andrew's handling ova. He has two children of his own and jokes that he does not know how they were conceived.

Leaning over a microscope, his white coat flapping open at the back, Trounson says: 'The first three were probably the best eggs. If anything this one had another four hours to go before it ovulated from the ovary; the others should have gone in the next hour or so.'

Illuminated from underneath, the human egg is merely a tiny blob of jelly; a single cell buoyed up by the sticky mass in which it floated in the follicle.

In June last year, 44-year-old Len Brennan stood over this microscope looking at an egg just taken from his wife Jan. It was the couple's third effort at conceiving a child with the help of science, and like the previous two, doomed to failure. They had to wait until October for success.

Len had a strict Catholic upbringing in the Yarram area of Victoria, but now rarely goes to church. He speaks of his glimpse down the microscope with reverence. 'I saw Jan's egg three minutes after it was picked up,' he says. 'It is a funny feeling looking at not even a new born infant but . . . the basis of life, I guess. To know your child before the egg is even fertilized would be a truly intimate thing.'

On that occasion Len sat with Jan as she came out of the anaesthetic to answer her first question: 'Did they get an egg?' In August and November of 1979, John Leeton had failed to find any eggs. This time the answer was 'Yes.'

A few days later they left the hospital and decided to call in at St Patrick's Cathedral where they sat for a few minutes drawing strength from the surroundings. Jan wished over and over to herself that the handful of cells — still too small to see with the naked eye — would grow into the child she wanted but could never have.

She says, 'You hoped that once you got a fertilized egg inside your womb, that you could have some sort of control of it. You thought "stick in there". If only you directed nice maternal thoughts towards it maybe it would stay . . . It didn't.'

For Jan, now twenty-seven, the process started when she was nineteen and working as a veterinary nurse. She suffered sudden severe abdominal pain. A doctor prescribed liquid aspirin and sent her back to work. 'Eventually I went back to the doctor but even then I was going to go back to work that day. I am one of those crazies who always insists on going to work. There was probably a bit of stupidity involved and by that stage I had lost a lot of weight and was very ill.'

She was referred to a gynaecologist who had her admitted to hospital for an immediate operation. She had peritonitis which had spread through her abdomen infecting appendix and Fallopian tubes — a vital link between the ovaries and uterus. Tubes and appendix were removed and for twenty-four hours it was doubtful whether Jan would pull through. After a month in hospital she was discharged; well but unable to have children.

'I didn't realize the effect it would have on me in future,' Jan says. 'I was only nineteen, I wasn't married, and I wasn't thinking of having children. I remember one of the nurses told me: "Don't worry dear, you can always breed dogs".'

In some ways Jan feels she was luckier than many of the 700 couples who are on the Monash team's waiting lists at the Queen Victoria Medical Centre and St Andrew's. Many of these couples have been through years of diagnostic testing and operations; Jan at least knew that a baby was impossible.

'I am just someone with a disability, a handicap,' Jan says. 'Obviously there is nothing externally wrong, but it is a disablement. People I know say they understand how I feel, but if you are able to have children, you can't really understand. Until you can't have something you don't know what you are missing out on.'

Jan feels she always wanted to be a mother. Len's six children from a previous marriage spend little time in Melbourne and when they did Jan was more a sister to them than a step-mother. Now, after three years' involvement with the test-tube programme, the baby has come to be vital to the couple's future.

'We have a total involvement with each other and this baby is an expression of Len's love for me and my love for him,' she says.

Jan and Len live in a small weatherboard bungalow close to the Dandenong shopping centre. Jan smiles above the clutter, saying that Len's spare-time renovations have reached only as far as the living-room and what is soon to be the child's bedroom.

She was a diving instructor at Portsea in 1974 when Len, then a married, settled dairy farmer walked into her class. In 1975, Len left his wife and children, driving away from his farm with only his clothes and a Kombi van. His children meant a lot to him, but his marriage to Jan, which took place in 1977, meant more. At the time there was no hope they would ever have children of their own.

Back in 1979 when test-tube babies seemed in the realm of science fiction, Jan and Len visited John Leeton in his rooms in Richmond. He explained the workings of the Monash programme which began back in 1970 but held out little hope of success.

Jan says: 'We had adjusted to the fact that we couldn't have children. There were times when I was depressed, feeling that somehow you weren't a real woman unless you were fertile. But we had the diving and we went away a lot to ride motor bikes. We filled our lives with other things.'

Then the first test-tube baby, Louise Brown, was born at Oldham Hospital in England. Monash re-started its programme and Jan and Len were one of the first couples to be accepted for treatment. By the time Jan and Len heard of their third failure in 1980 the constant travelling to and from the city and the tension of the programme was telling on their relationship. Both felt emotionally drained, especially as other women were becoming pregnant on their first attempt.

'When someone else in the programme becomes pregnant, to be honest, you feel jealous,' Jan says. 'You would be pleased that the programme was working, but couldn't help thinking "Why not for me?"'

In September 1980 Jan and Len helped to start the In Vitro Fertilization Friends group, a support group for the women on the programme. Then in October she rang Sister Wood to tell her that her period had begun. Like most members of the team Sister Wood wears many hats; helping in theatre and in this case co-ordinating the visits of the 250 couples receiving treatment at any one time.

There were several trips to the hospital before day five of Jan's cycle, when she began taking clomiphene pills. On day twelve Jan packed her bag and for the fourth time drove with Len to the city and the Queen Victoria. Then began three-hourly urine tests to monitor her hormone levels and a daily mucous test looking for possible sources of infection.

On 28 October John Leeton recovered two eggs from Jan's stimulated ovaries, and Len was called in to give a sample of semen. Between 500 000 and 750 000 sperm were added to each egg in small glass dishes which give the process its name — in vitro fertilization means, literally, in glass. Test tubes are used in other parts of the operation.

The dishes were placed in an incubator which mimics the temperature and humidity of the Fallopian tubes, where sperm normally meet ovum. The live sperm swim round the dish until the effects of gravity bring them close to the egg which lies on the bottom. The sperm then undergo subtle changes which allow them to penetrate the egg. It is believed that the head of the sperm becomes porous and releases a chemical which dissolves the egg's protective coating.

Test-tube fertilization differs here from the natural situation. Only a tiny fraction of a man's sperm will survive the arduous swim from the vagina to the Fallopian tubes. Only a handful, or at most 100, would be in the vicinity of the egg when it is fertilized. In the glass dish, the egg is surrounded by thousands of sperm. Reducing the number of sperm usually means the egg will not be fertilizied.

As soon as one sperm penetrates to the jelly-like centre of the egg, a granular barrier forms which blocks the advance of other sperm. After about twelve hours a nucleus forms within the sperm and within the egg containing the genetic information from man and woman. These two nuclei fuse together twenty-four to twenty-six hours after penetration by the sperm. At thirty hours the cell splits into two identical but smaller cells. The second division into four cells takes place at forty hours.

At fifteen minutes past midnight on 30 October, John Leeton and his team reassembled at St Andrew's to re-implant two eggs in Jan Brennan's uterus. One of the eggs was at the two-cell stage and the other was made up of four identical cells.

Leeton inserted a catheter through Jan's vagina that reached exactly to her uterus. Then Trounson, working under a microscope, drew the two eggs into a syringe with a single millilitre of fluid and injected them into the catheter.

'It really is a blind technique,' Professor Leeton says. 'When we implant the embryo inside a drop of fluid we can't even see it. It is one of those funny things. We are never sure that the embryo is ending up exactly where we want it.'

To help keep Jan's mind off the implantation Sister Wood sat by the operating table, holding her hand and talking about 'anything and everything'. This time it was the outfit she had bought to wear to the Melbourne Cup.

The implanted embryo is a conglomeration of identical cells. In some cases they have to be physically held together to prevent their breaking up. In the uterine environment divisions continue, but it is only after 120 hours that differences start appearing in the cells.

A small section of the cells remain embryonic or unformed, while most change to form the cells of the placenta. If all goes well, these burrow into the uterine wall. Implantation takes place on the sixth or seventh day. The first signs of the formation of the foetus — such as the beginnings of heart cells — start on about day sixteen.

Jan went home and settled down to wait. Waiting worries most of the test-tube patients. They wait to be admitted to the programme; they wait for their period to begin; for hormone levels to rise; for theatres to be booked; to see if eggs fertilize; and then to see if embryos implant.

'I was at work when Jillian Wood rang me up and said: ''Are you sitting down? Try not to get too excited, but you are pregnant'','' Jan says. 'By then I was on cloud nine. I rang Len and told him I was pregnant. He said: ''Are you sure?'''

Later blood samples showed that Jan was pregnant with twins — one of only two twin pregnancies achieved so far. But after only seven weeks she began bleeding from the vagina. She went back to hospital with the thought that it had all come to nothing. An ultrasound scan showed that one twin was dead.

'I was terribly worried and frightened, not knowing if the other would miscarry or if it would keep going,' Jan says.

For the next few weeks, she did not make any sudden movements for fear of losing the remaining twin. Then at fourteen weeks she began to bleed again; again she made the trip to the Queen Victoria for a week in hospital.

Somehow, the baby survived; a month later it gave its first kick. That was 'a lovely feeling', Jan says.

The ethics of aiding nature

Professor Carl Wood was walking along Elizabeth Street when he saw the newspaper poster: 'Frozen Human Embryos.' Heart sinking, he bought a copy and read the front-page story. The tone was of muted horror.

'People somehow see us as élite scientists playing with human life,' Professor Wood said. 'But we don't see ourselves as interfering with human life; we are assisting in the creating of it.'

As chairman of Monash University's Department of Obstetrics and Gynaecology, he has guided eleven years of research on the problems of infertility which affects about 30 000 Australian couples. It was in 1970 that he saw the potential for transferring laboratory fertilization techniques from animal husbandry to people.

Throughout, the programme has been guided by two separate ethics committees whose job it is to weigh the arguments of those who see a spiritual value in a four-celled embryo, and the more pragmatic view of the biologist. Professor Wood was brought up an apostolic Catholic and emerged with a deep understanding of theological questions.

'I don't accommodate the orthodox Catholic view, but I accommodate virtually everybody else,' Professor Wood said. 'I don't know that the Catholic view is correct or that the biologist's view is correct, and I am not arrogant enough either theologically or intellectually to say that I could be correct.'

A high proportion of patients in the Monash programme are Catholics; in Belgium, a Catholic university has started its own laboratory fertilization clinic.

But Professor Wood characteristically listens to the view of the Catholic heirarchy in Melbourne. His desire for a consensus also spreads to his relationship with colleagues and from them to patients. Important decisions — such as the number of fertilized embryos to be implanted and whether others should be frozen for later use — are made by the patients in consultation with the doctors. The patients feel they are part of a team.

As Professor Wood takes a telephone call in his office at the Queen Victoria Medical Centre he motions with his hand towards an egg-shaped ceramic sculpture which stands on a shelf together with photographs of some of the successful parents from the test-tube programme. The sculptured egg is cut open with a jagged line and inside is a tiny baby, its arms protectively covering his head — the gift of a Belgian potter.

On the wall next to his desk is a large white board showing a crude drawing of a woman's torso complete with details of sexual anatomy. Opposite is a large painting of a female nude with enormous buttocks painted in bright pastel colours. Patients would see both on their way to the small examination room.

Professor Wood was working on the musculature of the foetus when he switched scientific direction in 1970. Today he says he must have been a dreamer to think he could succeed where other 'better' scientists said he would fail. He says that to work on the programme one has to be an idealist, a workaholic, and prepared to try the unorthodox.

There were early suggestions to begin a monkey colony to test the procedures. That would have been a very expensive procedure. Using human volunteers would be more efficient and far more likely to bring results.

The Monash scientists attempted their first IVF in 1973 and another twenty to fifty attempts were made each year until 1978. On 25 July 1978 Louise Brown, the world's first test-tube baby was born in Britain to be followed on 14 January 1979 by Alastair Montgomery.

Success came to Melbourne on 23 June 1980 when Candice Reed was born in the Royal Women's Hospital. The Royal Women's group led by Mr Ian Johnston then split away from the Monash team after personality differences.

Professor Wood's group hit the news again on 10 March 1981 when a baby known only as Victoria was born at St Andrew's Hospital. In quick succession followed Carla Polson, an unnamed girl, twins Stephen and Amanda Mays, Sharna, an unnamed boy, David, Allison Arnastaukas and now Len and Jan Brennan's child . . . all except David, to Monash University's twenty-five-member team.

Professor Wood believes that the Monash team is now on a scientific par with the pioneering team of Steptoe and Edwards who operate a £1500 a time private clinic in Britain. While the British group has been criticized for withholding scientific information, Professor Wood's group has passed its techniques on to scientists around the world.

Lately Monash University has taken to issuing bulletins with birth scores such as 'Monash, 8; Rest of the World, 2.' The university has virtually supported the programme single-handed and at a cost of more than $1 million. Still, Professor Wood is embarrassed at suggestions that his team is ahead of the world: 'People see us as being ahead because they want us to be ahead. But I don't see us as any more than neck and neck.'

Professor Wood says his team's real successes have come in applying fertility pills to make ovulation more precise and more productive; the development of a vacuum needle which now allows a 90 per cent egg pick-up rate; and showing that pre-incubation of the egg improves the rate of growth of the embryo.

The latest advance has been to store embryos in a deep freeze for use later. This avoids the risk of more egg pick-up operations which must be done under general anaesthetic. Professor Wood sees the use of donor eggs as a next step. Donor semen has already resulted in one of the test-tube pregnancies and is commonly used in artificial insemination programmes.

The ethics committees have recommended against using surrogate mothers. Professor Wood has no personal objection to allowing one woman to carry a baby for another, if there is a good medical reason. But while fifty couples in the programme could perhaps employ the services of a surrogate mother, he feels the issue has not been discussed enough.

'At the moment we have got enough on our plate,' he said. 'The speed of change in this area has to be kept at a level that people can understand and accept. If too much happens too quickly, then people may not agree; you could lose the whole box and dice by going too fast.'

Professor Wood says the women in the programme are desperate to have a baby for various reasons, but behind it all is an innate wish to procreate. Many have spent a considerable part of their adult life attempting to cure their infertility.

'If I were in their position — I can't imagine being a woman anyway — I don't know that I would have that degree of endurance,' he said.

3 An Ethical Approach to IVF and ET: What ethics is all about

Helga Kuhse

Life is short, and Art long; opportunity is fleeting, experiment perilous, and judgment difficult.

Hippocrates

. . . and I say again that daily to discourse about virtue, and of those other things about which you hear me examining myself and others, is the greatest good of man, and that the unexamined life is not worth living, you are still less likely to believe me.

Socrates in Plato's *Apology*

'The unexamined life is not worth living.' With these words, Socrates — contemporary of Hippocrates and the first great moral philosopher of Western civilization — stated the creed of reflective men and women and set the task for ethics: to seek, with the help of reason, a consistent and defensible approach to life and its moral dilemmas.

Ethical inquiry is important to us when we are unsure of the direction in which we are heading. Like philosophy, it thrives on self-doubt. Athens after the death of Pericles and England after the death of Charles I are good examples. So is our time.

'New philosophy calls all in doubt,' wrote John Donne in the wake of the Copernican Revolution and of Charles I's violent death, suggesting that new thoughts had challenged old practices.[1] Today, new practices in the biomedical sciences are challenging old thoughts: 'New medicine calls all in doubt.'

Few moral convictions are more deeply ingrained than that of the sanctity of life. If plausible once, however, the view that life is a 'sacred process' (initiated, sustained, and finally halted by God) is now more difficult to maintain.[2] Recent advances in the biomedical sciences allow us to intervene in, and sometimes take control of, the processes of life and death. Not only can death, quite often, be kept waiting by the bed or machine, doctors and scientists can now also intervene in, indeed, initiate the process of life: cloning and recombination of DNA are two examples; IVF and ET another.

It is not surprising, then, that in the wake of these revolutionary developments bioethics is flourishing. Despite the obvious enthusiasm of philosophers to take a stand on many complex moral issues in the biomedical sciences, however, a curious scepticism pervades the enterprise. Take the comments by a dean of an Australian Medical School on the teaching of medical ethics:

Like any other lifelong clinical teacher I have firm views about such topics as euthanasia, continuing severe pain, acceptable and unacceptable risks of various treatments, the appropriate use of life support systems and numerous other matters of this sort which I discuss with my colleagues, assistants, and students but would not wish to teach dogmatically since much depends on the religious and ethical views which they may have and which also must command my respect.[3]

The paragraph suggests that although ethics is not a matter of dogmatism, it is a matter of personal preference or choice, something one cannot — or should not — argue about. Then there is another attitude, implied in a recent newspaper article by B. A. Santamaria, that ethical inquiry is useless unless those investigating bioethical issues have been '. . . endowed with authority by Almighty God [or] the Prime Minister . . .'[4]

IVF and ET raise many difficult moral issues. If the above conceptions about the nature of ethics were correct, however, discussion of these issues would either be futile (because morality is a matter of personal choice or opinion) or superfluous (because morality is what a divine or secular authority says it is).

In this chapter I shall argue that ethics is not simply a matter of personal preference or choice; that it depends neither on divine nor secular authority, and that reason and rational argument have a place in ethical inquiry. In other words, I want to suggest that it is not only possible but necessary to inquire into the ethics of such practices as IVF and ET: it is necessary because the fact that we *can* do something does not mean that we *ought* to do it. But if we want to show that the practice is either ethically acceptable or unacceptable, we have to provide reasons which go beyond personal opinion and the unquestioned acceptance of divine or secular authority.

How, then, can we approach ethical issues such as IVF? Although it would be tempting to plunge straight into a discussion of some of the moral problems as we see them, this approach would not be wholly satisfactory. We may find ourselves arguing about problems *within* ethics, without knowing what ethics is *about*, without having shown that ethics is a study in its own right. In other words, before we can debate questions within ethics, we must show that ethical argument is possible, that ethical judgements are something more than the expression of personal feelings, the dictates of authorities, or the codes of the societies in which we live.

The Nature of Ethics

Ethics is both ubiquitous and inescapable. Wherever people are living together, there is ethics: conduct is classified as 'right' or 'wrong'; standards are set. Ethics is part of the human condition.

To recognize that ethics is part of the human condition is one thing, however; to understand the nature of ethics is another. Here the basic question is whether ethics *has* a particular nature or whether it has as many natures as there are different human societies, or perhaps even different individuals who choose a particular ethics for themselves.

Ever since systematic Western philosophy had its beginning with Thales more than 2500 years ago, the question of the nature of ethics has been debated. So far, there is no ultimate agreement. 'Might it not follow', wrote the German philosopher Arthur Schopenhauer, 'from a retrospective glance at the main attempts to find a sure basis of morals for more than 2000 years that there is no natural morality at all that is independent of human institutions?'[5]

Even if we agree that there is no 'natural morality', however, just as there is no 'natural human being' in Rousseau's sense because both are also the products (and the producers!) of human institutions, of culture, this does not mean that ethics does not have an underlying nature. I want to suggest that it has and that the nature of ethics (Latin *natura* = 'birth', 'origin', 'character') is the rational element inherent in ethical thinking.

Before elaborating on the role of reason in ethics, it will be necessary to show why ethics is not synonymous with the dictates of divine or secular authorities, and why it is not simply a matter of personal attitudes.

Ethics and Authority

In the development of Western ethical thinking, the appeal to authority has been widespread. Historically, such claims have often been made on behalf of two types of authority: religious teachings or social practices, in the words of Santamaria: 'Almighty God or the Prime Minister'. I shall deal with ethics based on religion first.

It is often thought that ethics cannot survive without religion. In the words of Ivan Karamazov, if God is dead, then everything is permitted. But is it?

For hundreds of years, religious teachings provided a bulwark against ethical scepticism: '. . . God gives . . . content to the good . . . The good is what God rewards and the bad what he punishes.'[6] Today, religion — and with it a foundation of ethics on the will of God — is no longer universally accepted. This means that theological ethics has only a limited appeal. But philosophical ethics, in contrast to faith-based ethics, addresses a universal audience, not a particular sub-group. Moreover, a profound problem, first raised by Socrates in Plato's *Euthyphro*, is posed for anyone who wants to explain the nature of ethics in terms of the will of God. The question raised by Socrates is simply this: is a thing good because it is loved by the gods, or is it loved by the gods because it is good? This is not just a sophistical play with words. If 'good' were simply synonymous with 'loved by the gods', then goodness would be entirely arbitrary. Had the gods deemed to love torture, then torture would have been good. But to agree that torture would then have been good, makes morality entirely arbitrary; to deny that it would have been good presupposes the existence of ethical standards independent of the love, or will, of gods.[7]

In the light of this, many religious thinkers have given up the claim that ethics depends on theology of any sort; rather, they often agree that the basic principles of ethics must be defensible on non-religious grounds. In other words, they meet ethics on its own ground, that of reason. And that is, as we shall see, also the basis on which Ivan Karamazov would have to debate the principle that 'everything is permitted'.

It is obvious that the argument against identifying ethics with the will of God also applies in the case of a secular authority, such as the Prime Minister where, for many of us, non-identifiability would have an immediate, intuitive plausibility.

There is, however, another view which identifies ethics not with the dictates of a secular or divine authority but with the customs and practices of particular societies. Anthropologists and sociologists have shown that moral standards differ from culture to culture, and the claim has often been made that ethics is synonymous with group approval. As the sociologist W. G. Sumner put it at the beginning of this century: 'We shall find proof that ''immoral'' never means anything but contrary to the mores of the time and place . . . the ''right'' way is the way which the ancestors used and which has been handed down.'[8]

Most of us could give many examples to show that moral standards differ from culture to culture: the Moslems practice polygamy; the Jains will not eat meat; the Hopi are oblivious to animal suffering; the Eskimos allow first-born daughters to die of exposure.

On the Continent, Marxist and Freudian theories have added grist to the relativists' mills. Both views have one thing in common, the claim that human beings are 'conditioned', that their moral responses are determined either by their place in the economic system, or by familial relationships. If these claims were true, ethics would be superfluous. It would be swallowed up by either the study of political economy or psychoanalysis. (There is also a more recent contender, sociobiology, according to which 'the time has come for ethics to be removed temporarily from the hands of the philosopher and biologicized'.[9])

This way of thinking about ethics has been very influential. But is it correct? If our moral views were really determined by the economic system or by familial relationships, it is difficult to explain how the very proponents of such views can, themselves, raise questions about morality which have not been determined by, say, their position in the economic system.

Marx is the best example. Although a member of a particularistic class society, he was able to advance a universalistic view of ethics and society. But if this is possible because, as Marx suggests, consciousness can, at times, be 'further advanced than contemporary empirical relationships', it is difficult to see how consciousness could also have been *determined* by those very same empirical relationships.

We may be conditioned but not inescapably so. We still can, and do, ask whether the practices of our society, class, or family, are right or wrong as, indeed, did Marx.[10]

And we can do the same regarding the moral codes of other societies. That different societies have different moral codes proves nothing in itself. There is also disagreement between cultures about non-moral matters. Some people believed that the earth was a flat disc, others that it was a great ball resting on the back of a turtle, and some that looking at your mother-in-law caused disease. If we do not, from such disagreement, draw the conclusion that there is no truth or falsity to geography or medicine, why conclude from ethical disagreement that there is no truth or falsity to ethics? Societies, like individuals, can be mistaken in their ethical judgements as is perhaps best demonstrated by citing the example of Nazi Germany.

Contemporary philosophers generally reject the claim that ethics is relative in these senses. The claim of relativity, however, survives in a different form. In this view, which goes back to Hume, ethical judgements do not belong to the class of statements called cognitive, which can be verified as true or false; rather, ethical judgements are emotional expressions of approval or disapproval, or are merely prescriptions for action.

On these 'emotivist' or 'prescriptivist' views, variations and conflict between moral utterances are relative to the varying conditions that give rise to such feelings, attitudes, or prescriptions. Why do we use ethical language? We use it to express our attitudes and needs, and to manipulate the behavioural dispositions in our hearers. We do this because we care about our feelings and attitudes and care about what people do.

If we accept this view of ethics, often described as 'subjectivist', does this mean that one ethical judgement is as good as another? I think not. Even if there is, as the subjectivists suggest, no separate realm of ethical facts and values that exists independently of us, this does not mean that there is no room for argument, that one ethical judgement is as good as another. Contemporary subjectivists, such as J. L. Mackie and J. J. C. Smart, agree that reason has some role to play in ethics: arguments in support of moral judgements can be criticized, shown to be adequate or inadequate, on a number of grounds. In other words, moral problems are amenable to solution by rational methods.[11]

Ethics and Rationality

To be tenable, ethical judgements must pass two minimal tests: they must be consistent and in some sense universal. Let me deal with consistency first.

Inconsistency is a fatal flaw in any argument, including ethical argument. If we can detect an inconsistency in someone's view, we feel that we have dealt it a mortal blow. Even David Hume, to whom modern subjectivism can be traced, employed this device in his famous argument against the prohibition of suicide. His argument was this: if the objection to suicide is that we must not cut short our lives because by doing so we interfere in the 'sacred process' of life, that is, usurp the prerogative of God to give and take life then, surely, we usurp His prerogative no less when we deliberately lengthen our lives. As Hume put it: 'If I turn aside a stone which is falling upon my head, I disturb the course of nature, and I invade the peculiar province of the Almighty by lengthening out my life beyond the point which . . . he had assigned it.'[12]

This means that the objection to suicide must either be based on something other than the usurpation argument or, if it isn't, not only the shortening but also the lengthening of life must be forbidden. We must stand still and wait for the stone to hit. Those who claim that we interfere in the 'sacred process' when we shorten life, but not when we lengthen it, are being inconsistent.

A similar argument may have implications for the debate over IVF. If the objection to IVF is based simply on the view that it involves us in 'playing God' because we deliberately initiate life, then someone may suggest that we are also 'playing God' when we deliberately refrain from initiating life. To put it somewhat differently, an objector may be pressed to explain why we play God only when we do something but not when we deliberately do nothing.

Inconsistencies and confusions appear in many guises, even in the concepts we employ in our ethical arguments. This is why it is sometimes impossible to make progress in an ethical impasse until we have clarified the concepts that are crucial to the debate.

Take the abortion debate, for example. The most fundamental question raised by abortion is the moral status of the foetus. This is, of course, also the fundamental question raised by IVF if not all embryos are implanted into the womb but are discarded or frozen at some stage after fertilization has occurred. It is not surprising, then, that it seems scarcely possible to take a stand on the debate over IVF without having come to grips with the issue that is at the heart of the abortion debate: whether all human life is of the same quality or kind and sacrosanct from the moment of conception. Here, pro-abortionists may want to argue that the concept 'human being' spans two different kinds of life: mere biological life and the life of a person in the sense of a rational or self-conscious being. Hence, the argument may hinge on what we mean by a 'human being' and by a 'person' and what particular qualities or attributes are morally relevant to the wrongness of killing. Confusion over the meanings of these terms could lead to conclusions about abortion that we will consider indefensible once the concepts have been clarified.

There is also another test which an ethical judgement must pass: it must be impartial or universal. If I suggest that a certain action is right or wrong, good or bad, I am committed to taking the same view about any relevantly similar action. For example, if I say that it is right for me to make a lying promise because I want to avoid mild inconvenience, but wrong for you to do so, then you can demand a reason in support of my view. If my position is to be ethically acceptable, then I cannot point only to the advantages that lying brings me. As Hume puts it, anyone seeking to justify his conduct ethically must 'depart from his private and particular situation and must choose a point of view common to him with others'.[13] In other words, conduct is ethical only if it is in some sense impartial, if it can be defended from a universal point of view.

The idea that ethical conduct must in some sense be universal has a long history. It finds expression in the ancient golden rule, 'Do unto others as you would have them do unto you', in Kant's famous formulation of the categorical imperative, 'Act only on that maxim through which you can at the same time will that it should become a universal law', in the universal prescriptivism of the Oxford philosopher R. M. Hare, and in the universal pragmatics of the contemporary German Marxist Jürgen Habermas, who sees 'universalization as the only principle in which practical reason [that is, ethics] expresses itself'.[14]

This means that even if we have severed the link between religion and ethics, even if life cannot be seen as a 'sacred process', not everything is permitted as Ivan Karamazov thought, at least not if we want to act ethically. Ethics demands that we go beyond our individual standpoint, beyond what benefits us and our family or group, and that we adopt the 'universal point of view'.

The Ethical Approach to IVF and ET

To demand that ethics be in some sense consistent and universal is one thing; to derive from these formal requirements an ethical theory which will be able to guide our conduct is another. The point is this: quite different ethical theories can be derived from the formal aspects of ethical thinking. Kantianism and utilitarianism are perhaps the most familiar examples, but there are many others. What is more, none has met with general acceptance.

What, then, are we to do? How can we approach the question of IVF, and how will we know that our approach is an ethical one?

Let me begin by saying that an approach comes within the realm of the ethical if it is backed by *reasons* acceptable from an impartial or universal point of view, that is, if its proponents are prepared to offer supportive ethical arguments for their view. For example, if people were to object to IVF on the basis that this practice separates 'lovemaking' from 'babymaking' and were to add that this separation is wrong because it is an intrusion into the 'sacred process' of life, they have provided a reason for their view. Even if we regard the justification as ultimately inadequate, the attempt to provide a reason of a universal kind brings the approach within the realm of the ethical.

We can go further than this. We saw that the ethical approach must be consistent and universal. If the 'sacred process' objection to IVF were found, for example, to be inconsistent with the general curative approach of medicine to disease (which does, after all, constitute an intervention into the 'sacred' or 'natural' process), this might be a reason for rejecting it.

More generally, we might agree with Socrates that the ethical approach requires us to examine critically our lives and our practices. What is more, we must recognize that this is a continuing process. The uncritical retention of ethical tenets that may have served us well in a different time and under different circumstances is equivalent to the 'unexamined life', which Socrates thought less than human. This means that morality may have to be re-fashioned when our framework for action is changed. As J. L. Mackie notes, we cannot brush this aside by pointing out that morality 'has been made already, long ago. It may well need to be in part remade'.[15]

The point is not only that 'new medicine *calls all in doubt*'; there is, as the American bioethicist Robert Veatch notes, 'something about the life and death issues raised by advanced medical technology which *forces* us to re-think all the basic problems of morality'.[16] We are literally forced to re-think many basic problems of morality because adherence to traditional tenets can often be bought only at the price of inconsistency.

To give just two crude examples: there seems to be something profoundly wrong with holding the view that all human life, regardless of its quality or kind, has the same sanctity or value, and yet discontinuing artificial life support in the case of a permanently comatose patient, while indefinitely continuing artificial life support in the case of a patient who is not permanently comatose. Does not the difference in treatment suggest that we regard the quality of life of a patient as morally relevant? Similarly, the sanctity-of-life view fits poorly with the practice of not operating on a Down's syndrome baby with an intestinal obstruction, thus 'letting it die', when the same operation would be performed on a baby born with an intestinal obstruction but not afflicted with Down's syndrome.

One way of overcoming inconsistencies such as these is to bring our beliefs in line with our actions by critically examining, for example, the sanctity-of-life view. This means that inconsistencies can be motivating factors in their own right, that is, have a profound influence on our ethical views. On this both Marxist and non-Marxist philosophers agree. Habermas puts it this way: 'Normative structures can be overturned directly through cognitive dissonance between secular knowledge — expanded with the development of the forces of production — and the dogmatics of traditional world views.'[17] Singer, in his less convoluted prose, makes the same point: '. . . if we sense an inconsistency in our beliefs and actions, we will try to do something to eliminate the sense of inconsistency, just as when we feel hungry we will try to do something to eliminate our hunger', and one way of doing this is to make 'our beliefs and actions both true and consistent'.[18]

This has implications for the revolutionary development in medicine of being able to separate sexual and reproductive activities. Not only can we, through the development of effective contraceptive devices, now engage in sexual intercourse without producing children, we can now also, through the development of IVF and ET, produce children without engaging in sexual intercourse. The question is, though, whether we can, in the light of these new abilities, also continue to see the moment of conception as sacrosanct and as the beginning not only of human life but also of its inviolability. The point is this: predictions are that the next few years will see not only the perfection of IVF techniques but also the possibility of partho-genesis (producing off-spring from unfertilized eggs) and cloning. This means that not only every fertilized egg but every unfertilized egg, indeed, each cell is a potential embryo and hence a potential human being.

Does this mean we are doing something wrong each time we do not sustain an unfertilized ovum, each time we do not help a cell to fulfil its new potential? I think not. But if we take the view that it is not wrong to prevent potential human life from becoming actual in the case of cloning and parthogenesis, we may be forced to abandon the view that the wrongness of abortion and the wrongness of dis-carding embryos in the course of IVF procedures lies in the foetus' or embryo's potential. If these practices are wrong, their wrongness must lie elsewhere.

If I am correct in this, biomedical advances such as IVF may trigger a change in our traditional moral attitudes. 'But', the per-ceptive reader may interject, 'this means that ethics is relative after all!' Yes, but only in a superficial sense. Let me explain:

If we are not absolutists, that is, if we do not adhere to our moral principles regardless of the consequences, we will agree that actions that are right in one situation can be wrong in another because of their consequences. Take the well-worn example that it is wrong to lie. Would it also be wrong to lie if by doing so we could save the lives of ten Jews hiding from the Gestapo in Nazi Germany? Hardly. Similarly, the medical dictum that a doctor should prolong life if he or she can. Again, this would be the right action under normal circumstances. But take the case of a baby born with Lesch-Nyham disease. This is a metabolic disorder which affects the central nervous system. It is characterized by absence of co-ordination, mental re-tardation, aggressive behaviour, and compulsive self-mutilation, which begins the moment the baby cuts its first tooth. The disease is at present incurable, and the child inevitably dies in early infancy. Should the doctor always prolong the life of a Lesch-Nyham infant? Once again, I think not.

We may thus agree that certain rules, such as 'do not lie', 'always prolong life', are relative to time and place, that their rightness or wrongness depends on the particular circumstances of the situation. But the acceptance of this surface relativity says nothing about the truth or falsity of such principles under certain specified circum-stances (such as Lesch-Nyham disease), or against more fundamental principles, such as the utilitarian principle 'an action is right in proportion as it tends to produce happiness and wrong as it tends to produce unhappiness', or the deontological principle 'an action is morally right if it is the action required by a duty which is at least as strong as any other duty in the circumstances'. Although fundamental principles such as these may not change with time and place, it seems that some of the rules that have been fashioned to help us achieve those ends do.

This has implications for the sanctity-of-life ethic and, by extension, for IVF and ET, as well as for a whole host of other developments in the biomedical sciences. To put it bluntly, in the light of these developments, the sanctity-of-life view may have outlived its usefulness. In making this comment, I do not stand isolated. Many philosophers, theologians, and doctors agree that the time has come to replace the sanctity-of-life ethic by a quality-of-life approach.[19]

Why? Because the traditional sanctity-of-life ethic is no longer able to guide our actions in an unequivocal way. Take the comments of Dr David Hamburg, a member of the Ethics Advisory Board, appointed by the American Department of Health, Education, and Welfare to investigate the ethics of IVF: 'Much of the discussion . . . has revolved [around] a basic value of our society, the sanctity of life. I find myself genuinely perplexed, deeply perplexed, about how to apply that fundamental value in this context.'[20]

This perplexity is not surprising. If we understand the sanctity-of-life concept as a 'sacred process', we have to explain why we may interfere in the process when prolonging life but not when shortening it. Or, in the case of IVF, why it should be wrong to deliberately initiate the process, but not wrong deliberately not to initiate it. Or, if we understand the sanctity-of-life concept in the traditional Catholic sense of an absolute prohibition against the intentional termination of innocent human life, no matter what its stage of development or its quality, we have to defend ourselves not only against the charge of being 'speciesist' (something no better than a racist or sexist) but also explain the inconsistency that arises when we are permitted,[21] despite this absolute rule, to cease treatment which would have prolonged life, indeed, to turn off the respirator which sustains the life of a permanently comatose, not dead, patient. And the examples could go on.

But if the sanctity-of-life doctrine has lost its central position in our value system, if it can no longer guide our actions in an unequivocal way, does this, once again, mean that 'everything is permitted'? More particularly, can we conclude that IVF and ET are morally acceptable practices? We cannot draw this conclusion, and not only because the points I have been making are only sketches, rather than fully blown arguments, but also because even if objections to IVF based on some versions of the sanctity-of-life view cannot be sustained, there may be other objections which can.

Let me mention one possible objection which is problematic not only because it relies on notoriously difficult predictions, but also because it poses a dilemma for ethical theory itself. We may agree that there is nothing intrinsically wrong with the practice of IVF, with the separation of reproductive and sexual activities, that there is no moral difference between discarding surplus human embryos and deliberately not creating them in the first place, and yet objecting to such practices on the ground of their possible consequences: the spectre of the Brave New World haunts the imagination.

The point is this: the new techniques of being able to initiate life outside the body bring with them other possibilities as well. They bring with them the possibility of manipulating the genetic structure of this budding human life; and the prospects of genetic engineering and cloning. Once again, there may be nothing wrong with the practices as such. On the contrary, we may be able to employ recombinant DNA techniques to eliminate many of the more than 3000 known chromosomal or genetic disorders, and the children who will be born following genetic 'surgery' may be glad that these techniques were available to make their lives better than they would have been. However, there is also the other side of the coin. In 1979, Dr Jonathan King, Professor of Microbiology at the Massachusetts Institute of Technology in Boston, discussed the possibilities of genetic engineering: 'Scientists may soon be able to provide us with an addition to the human race: a class of three-armed people all owned by a private corporation. Their food supply would probably come first, four-legged chickens, for example, with the obvious advantage of two extra drum-sticks.'[22] The chickens were still science fiction in 1979. But now, in 1981, they have become reality. Newspapers reported recently that the first four-legged chicken had been produced and was doing well. At the moment, the three-armed people are still in the realm of science fiction. But for how long? And if we *could* develop them, what moral arguments could we put up to counter such developments?

Here we return to the beginning. The Copernican Revolution meant not only that the earth had lost its central position in the universe, but also that the Great Chain of Being had been broken once and for all. As John Donne put it, with the sun lost and the cosmos 'all in pieces', 'Prince, Subject, Father, Son are things forgot'. And just as Thomas Hobbes and John Locke were compelled to work out anew the meanings of authority and subjection, so may we, faced with a revolution in the biomedical sciences, have to work out anew the meanings of life and death, what it is that gives special value to human life and when, and for whom, death is an evil.

Hippocrates is correct: judgement is difficult and experiment perilous. And yet, and because of it, answers must be found. The uncritical acceptance of the 'new science', no less so than the uncritical acceptance of the 'old morality' are constituents of the 'unexamined life'. How can we examine our lives and our practices? Through discourse and argumentation. As Habermas puts it, once called into question, truth claims can be resolved only through the force of the better argument, through an analysis of the notion of providing rational grounds.[23]

And that, I suppose, is what this book and the debate on IVF and ET is ultimately all about, as, indeed, is ethics.

4 For and Against: The essence of the arguments as they appeared in the press

Life Rally told Embryos may be Killed

Tony Harrington

The Right to Life Association yesterday called on the Queen Victoria Hospital to close its in vitro test-tube baby programme.

The association's state president, Mrs Margaret Tighe, told a rally of about 10 000 anti-abortionists in the Treasury Gardens that doctors were now in a position to destroy twelve excess embryos stored in a laboratory freezer at the hospital.

She called on doctors to concentrate their research on curing infertility instead of creating embryos from fertilized human eggs outside the womb.

Three Melbourne babies have successfully been delivered under the in vitro programme in which doctors thaw the embryos and implant them in women to develop normally.

Several leftover embryos were frozen and stored for future test-tube baby programmes after researchers decided to use fertility drugs on some women as a cheaper way of achieving a greater success. Mrs Tighe said the embryos might be destroyed.

'In Australia doctors are killing thousands of unborn children, yet here they are going to extraordinary lengths to create new ones. It's really upside down.'

Mrs Tighe said Australian doctors had done little or no research into ways of repairing blocked Fallopian tubes, although an American doctor had claimed an 80 per cent success rate in overcoming the problem.

'Our doctors should be concentrating on this, not playing around with human life,' she said.

Mrs Tighe said the association would take an active interest in next year's state election, concentrating on marginal seats.

She defended the association's move to make abortion an election issue as the only effective way of publicizing the cause. Former Liberal MHR Mr Barry Simon had lost his seat of McMillan at last year's federal election only because of the group's campaign against him, she said.

The only disruption to the demonstration was the chanting of about 100 members of the International Socialists Movement who, separated by two lines of police, criticized the Right to Life Association during the Treasury Gardens rally.

They claimed the association was concerned only with unborn children but not with the right to life of people killed by governments in countries including Chile and El Salvador.

'These people are being very emotive by saying they want to protect unborn lives,' said one of the socialist speakers. 'But have they ever demonstrated against toxic waste dumps or 2,4,5-T?'*

Frozen Embryos Preserve Life

Carl Wood, W. A. W. Walters and *John F. Leeton*

We wish to comment on the report (13/4) 'Life Rally Told Embryos May Be Killed.'*

The whole point of freezing embryos is to preserve life, not destroy it. The advice of the Queen Victoria Medical Centre Ethics Committee, which includes a Roman Catholic theologian, was to freeze embryos in an attempt to preserve life. On occasions, fresh embryos cannot be transferred to the uterus because of technical difficulties or because an excess of embryos is available. Rather than destroy the embryo, we are attempting to preserve it by freezing and to transfer the embryo back to the uterus at a more favourable time.

*This news report and the following letters all appeared in the *Age* newspaper 1981

At no time, as Mrs Tighe is quoted as saying, do we intend to destroy the embryo.

The system of freezing has great potential. It is very common in the natural system of conception for embryos to be destroyed. Only about 25 per cent to 30 per cent of fertilizations end up as live, healthy babies. By developing the freezing technique, it may be possible in the future to save some of the normal embryos (many early abortions may be abnormal embryos) that are destined to be destroyed by nature.

Timely collection and freezing of embryos threatened by abnormal environmental circumstances, such as fever or bleeding from the uterus, may enable re-transfer of normal embryos under more favourable circumstances later. In this way, some natural abortions may be prevented in the future. How can Mrs Tighe rally her anti-abortion movement against a medical group which is aiming to create or preserve new life?

Mrs Tighe mentions that Australian doctors have done little or no research into ways of repairing blocked Fallopian tubes, and quoted an American doctor who claimed an 80 per cent success rate in overcoming the problem. Her facts are incorrect. Microsurgery has been developed in Australia to improve the results of tubal repair.

Mr B. O'Brien, head of the microsurgical unit at St Vincent's Hospital, taught Mr P. Paterson, Dr B. Downing and Professor Wood microsurgery, so that we could apply these techniques to improve methods of surgical repair. This group was the first in Australia and, along with an English group, was the first in the world to publish results of human tubal microsurgery.

As a result, we have been asked to speak at a number of symposiums in other countries on the new surgical techniques and to write chapters in overseas surgical textbooks. A number of Melbourne gynaecologists including those at the Royal Women's, St Vincent's, Mercy Maternity, Western General, Essendon, and Prince Henry's now practise microsurgery to improve the results of tubal surgery. The figure of 80 per cent success rate, quoted by Mrs Tighe, applies only to tubes that are little damaged and where the repair usually can be effective.

No one in the world has a success rate, which includes all patients with tubal disease, of more than 50 per cent. Because so many women have irreparably damaged tubes, the process of IVF has been developed. Because Mrs Tighe does not agree with a specific procedure, should other women who wish to become pregnant be deprived of the chance to become a mother?

Another attempt to overcome tubal infertility was pioneered in Melbourne. Mr O'Brien, Professor Wood, Dr I. McKenzie and Dr B. Downing, with the help of other surgeons and physicians, were the first in the world to report a human tube transplant done by microsurgical vascular techniques. This did not succeed, but led to Professor Wood being asked to speak in other countries, including France, Spain, and Italy, on the subject of tubal transplantation.

Difficulties in the use of potentially toxic anti-immune drugs for the treatment of a non life-threatening disease is holding up research in the area of tubal transplantation.

The work of Australian specialists in tube infertility hardly fits Mrs Tighe's alleged statements of 'little or no research' or 'our doctors should be concentrating on this' (tubal repair). The only threat to Australia maintaining a successful place in infertility research is that, as a result of Mrs Tighe misinforming the public about our objectives, practice and achievements, public and government support may be withheld.

Test-tube Baby Research involves Moral Questions

Sir Frank Little, Roman Catholic Archbishop of Melbourne

Professor Carl Wood states in his letter (18/4) that on the question of freezing human embryos the advice of the Queen Victoria Medical Centre Ethics Committee, which includes a Roman Catholic theologian, was to freeze embryos in an attempt to preserve life.

Such a statement can carry the implication that the Roman Catholic Church therefore approves of IVF. Some have so interpreted the professor's words.

I wish to correct that impression.

Within the context of the professor's letter, there are two main issues at stake.

He is writing of what should be done with an excess of living human embryos, for the existence of which his team has been responsible. The major alternatives appear to be either to destroy them (his own word) or freeze them. He argues that they should be frozen. Faced with the destruction of human life at that stage, one can understand his decision.

That is one issue.

The other issue, the very question of the morality of IVF, is the major one.

One must first ask whether Professor Wood and those associated with him had the moral right to embark on a procedure which placed them in the predicament of 'destruction or freezing'.

I understand that elsewhere reticence in this area of research is due to the fact that others are still seeking to come to terms with the moral issues.

One's heart goes out to those infertile couples who see this procedure as enabling them to achieve their desire for parenthood. That is understandable. One cannot but feel compassion for them.

But does the end justify the means?

The embryo must be regarded as a person, never as an object. Is the dignity of the human person fully expressed, and adequately safeguarded, in the so-called test-tube production of human life?

The moral questions associated with this issue are multiple and need much public discussion to prevent scientific action outstripping the moral principles on which it should be based.

Should we not commence with the fundamental principle: God has bound the transmission of human life to the conjugal sex act. If science helps only to accomplish the marital act or to continue a marital act already initiated, then there is no problem; but if science seeks to exclude or substitute the marital act, the scientific action is not licit.

Test-tube Babies have High Price

M. Tighe, president of the Right to Life Association

I write in response to Professors Wood, Walters and Leeton (18/4).

The point at issue is not the ability of Australian doctors to repair blocked Fallopian tubes, but rather the highly undesirable risks to human life that are inevitably involved in the IVF programme.

One might well ask what price in human life must be paid to produce one healthy test-tube baby?

Professor Jerome Lejeune, chairman of Genetics at Paris University, and famed for his discovery of the cause of Down's syndrome, has this to say of IVF: 'The people who started the technique said that it was to by-pass the obstacle of an obstructed tube. This is seemingly acceptable, but you have to know that it is, I would not say make-believe, but very close to it, because tubal obstruction can be treated by graft, by transplantation, by a lot of techniques which are evolving and which are much more promising and will interest many more women than IVF.'

All three professors protest that by freezing the 'left-over' embryos, they are in fact preserving life. At least while there is life, there is hope.

How did these twelve hapless frozen embryos come into existence? Dr Kovacs, one of the medical scientists in the in vitro team speaking on 'Nationwide' (6/4), said: 'It is a problem that has arisen as a by-product of the project and it wasn't one that was necessarily contemplated.'

Having created these unfortunate human 'by-products', the in vitro team is apparently going to seek guidance on their future from the self-styled bioethics committee at Monash University.

Professor Peter Singer, chairman of this bioethics committee assured us on 'Nationwide' (6/4) that if it was decided to destroy the embryos, it would after all be no different from an abortion.

Can Professors Wood, Walters and Leeton give us assurances that the frozen 'left-over' embryos will be implanted in their mothers in the near future? Can they also assure us that the utmost respect for human life pervades the whole in vitro programme?

One cannot surely be blamed for expressing concern about and opposition to the whole scheme given the record of the Queen Victoria Medical Centre. The hospital is listed in many municipal services guides as a place where 'late terminations of pregnancy are available'.

Further, one cannot surely be blamed for opposing the test-tube baby project when one considers that in vitro researchers Wood, Walters and Leeton also head the Obstetrics and Gynaecological Department of this hospital.

Medical Technology Threatens Women

M. Gladwin, senior tutor, Graduate Diploma in Women's Studies, Rusden State College, in association with P. Gowland, tutor in Feminist Philosophy, Council of Adult Education

It was with deep concern that I read of the pronouncements of the ethics committee of the Queen Victoria Medical Centre regarding the preservation of 'life' at conception by freezing fertilized embryos (the *Age*, 18/4). The questions to ask are: 'Does life begin in the test-tube' and 'Are Carl Wood *et al.* really clandestine members of the Right to Life Association?'

The claim that life begins at the moment of conception and therefore should be preserved has long been part of the rhetoric of reactionary forces in the community. This view has serious consequences for the right of women to control their reproductive processes. Carl Wood *et al.* have assumed the garb of arbiters of much debated philosophical questions as well as assuming instrumental control over life and death.

Until now one of the few recognized achievements of women was their ability to reproduce life in the womb. They now face the prospect of losing even the right to control their fundamental female processes.

Can we afford to invest in 'men of science' the right to make ethical judgements? What assurances do we have that these judgements will direct the development and application of new medical technology? The evidence to date seems to justify grave concern about the implications of this technology for women's lives.

For example, Professor Carl Wood and Gabor Kovacs support the use of Depo Provera (3/4) as a long-term contraceptive for young women despite the claims of its detrimental effects. Rather than a concern for 'the preservation of life', the history of the medical profession's involvement in birth-related technologies shows a serious disregard for the preservation of women's lives and well-being. This is evident in the suffering caused to women and their children by the use of inadequately researched drugs such as DES and Thalidomide and the illness and death brought about by the Dalkon Shield.

Furthermore, where the brain hormone LRF is used to 'cure' female infertility caused by 'stress, depression . . . (even long distance running)' (the *Age*, 28/2) shouldn't we be preventing the oppressive social conditions that give rise to this situation? Similarly, should the 'problem' of the childless couple be subjected to medical treatment rather than examining the social values which define infertility and childlessness as forms of deficiency and deprivation?

While not being insensitive to the distress of some women who cannot produce a child, we believe that a social rather than a surgical solution is possible. A socially responsible view of parenting, for example, would see it as a widely shared human experience.

Further control of women's reproductive processes should not be handed over to those who are unauthorized to make ethical decisions and who are blind to the real conditions of human beings in our society.

Researchers must have Reverence for Life

William Daniel

I would like to offer a comment on the letter of Professor Carl Wood (18/4) regarding the freezing of embryos in the IVF procedure.

He presents the freezing of embryos as an attempt to save them, rather than let them perish. 'On occasions fresh embryos cannot be transferred to the uterus because of technical difficulties or because an excess of embryos is available.'

The last clause quietly introduces and passes over what, to my mind, is the most controversial aspect of the procedure, ethically speaking. Why is 'an excess of embryos' available? Because the doctors have induced superovulation in the woman, have harvested a number of eggs, and then have fertilized them. It should not be referred to as one would refer to some unaccountable natural event. And they have done this with the clear understanding that it is most unlikely that more than one or two of them will ever be given the chance to develop in the uterus.

Professor Wood and his collaborators can honestly say that they do not intend to destroy the embryo. But they cannot deny that they do intend to fertilize more ova than they can ever hope to transfer. They cannot offer the chance of continued life to the surplus embryos.

We get admonitions from time to time on the irresponsibility of bringing more children into the world than we can (conveniently) care for. Now, there is at least a chance that a child born live into the world can get adequate care from some other source if the family cannot provide it. But what kind of responsibility is it towards the life we engender if we foresee that we cannot even offer it the chance to proceed beyond the first cell divisions?

Multiple fertilization with freezing of surplus embryos seems to me the typical approach of the well-meaning technologist. It would be quite possible for them to fertilize only one ovum and endeavour to get that to develop in the uterus. But it makes better technological sense to utilize all the material harvested. Here the keynote is 'utility' and 'material'. It cannot be reconciled with a proper reverence for human life in its beginnings.

If that reverence is lacking, IVF is blighted at the source, and will prove to be but the first step on the way to all the clever things that the genetic engineers and others have in store for us.

Puzzling Opposition to Test-tube Babies

Peter Singer

In her letter on the issue of IVF (27/4) Mrs Tighe of the Right to Life Association claims I said — in a recent 'Nationwide' interview — that if it were decided to destroy frozen embryos, this would be no different from an abortion.

Mrs Tighe's report of what I said is inaccurate. The statement I made was in reply to the question of whether it would be murder to destroy a frozen embryo, and my reply was that *at worst* it would be an abortion. I was not saying that the destruction of a frozen embryo is in fact equivalent to an abortion, but rather that by no stretch of the imagination could it be considered any *more* serious than an abortion.

I then went on to agree with Dr Kovacs when he pointed out that a more appropriate parallel would be not with an abortion which destroys an embryo several weeks along the process of development, but rather with the effect that some IUDs have. There is evidence that these devices often prevent pregnancy not by preventing conception, but rather by preventing the fertilized egg from implanting in the womb. The embryo is thus destroyed at the very earliest stage of its existence, as would be the case if the frozen embryos at the Queen Victoria Medical Centre were to be destroyed.

While I accept that the IVF programme raises significant ethical issues, it would be interesting if the Right to Life Association would explain why it has focussed its opposition on the possible destruction of these frozen embryos, while it is relatively silent about the use of IUDs which have the same effect.

Its opposition to the IVF programme is particularly puzzling in view of two facts: firstly, that the whole aim of the programme is to create human life — something that the Right to Life Association could be expected to support — and secondly, that the embryos in question would never even have existed, were it not for the efforts of the doctors Mrs Tighe is criticizing.

Respect for Life in Research

Carl Wood

The following are replies to recent letters.

Mrs Margaret Tighe (27/4).
In answer to her questions:

Six of the frozen embryos have already been implanted.

The utmost respect for human life pervades the whole in vitro programme. The Queen Victoria Medical Centre Clinic for termination of pregnancies has nothing to do with the IVF programme; the latter is organized by the Monash University Department of Obstetrics and Gynaecology with the assistance of the staff and administration of the Queen Victoria Medical Centre.

The in vitro researchers, Wood, Walters, and Leeton, do not head the Obstetric and Gynaecological Department of the Queen Victoria Medical Centre. There is a rotating chairman of the Division of Obstetrics and Gynaecology — Mr Arthur Day is the current chairman. Policy is determined by all members of the consultant staff, the university members of the hospital being in a minority.

The meaning of Dr Kovac's statement was not clear. Freezing was decided upon as a deliberate policy to preserve life and also as a technique which, in the future, may help other infertile women to have babies.

Professor Jerome Lejeune is wrong on two accounts. The IVF procedure is no longer very close to make-believe. Tubal grafts or transplantation have not yet produced one live healthy baby and therefore cannot be more promising as techniques. Once non-toxic drugs are available to prevent rejection, the situation may change.

Maree Gladwin and Patricia Gowland (27/4).

The decision to use IVF was a result of the medical ethic to relieve human suffering. The request for resolution came from women and men, and the technology developed from this. The ethical decisions are shared with the patients, both women and men, and the hospital ethics committee, consisting of both women and men. It is incorrect to say that women face the prospect of losing the right to control their fundamental female processes.

The natural system continues and the use of any artificial system depends upon the request from couples. 'Men of science' do not make ethical decisions — ethical decisions are shared with men and women, both in and outside science.

Community debate, such as presented by the concern expressed in your letter will contribute to the ethical considerations and help in determining the use or restriction of any new technology. However, I do not see the current technique as a threat to women.

The debate on Depo Provera is realistic. The current evidence suggests that, if a woman cannot tolerate or use other contraceptive methods, then Depo Provera is certainly more preferable than an unwanted pregnancy with the possibility of therapeutic abortion and so on. No method of contraception is without disadvantage. It is a matter of weighing evidence and people often differ in such matters.

I agree that social resolution of infertility is important, but it is not yet feasible. The doctor has a duty to care for individuals and, in seeking to resolve personal suffering from infertility, therapy is offered.

The disasters of Thalidomide and DES were due to serious errors in the selection of drugs, but weighed against the many advances made by the medical profession that have reduced maternal mortality and morbidity and perinatal mortality does not validate a charge that the medical profession has a 'serious disregard for the preservation of women's lives and well-being'.

William Daniel (28/4).   *Religions*

The basis of Father Daniel's letter is Roman Catholic teaching, that a two-cell embryo, which cannot be seen by the naked eye, is human life, and not potential human life. The law, biology, and other religious groups distinguish between human life according to its stage of development. It is unfair to assume others have no proper reverence because they do not follow Roman Catholic teaching and accord a different degree of reverence to a two-cell embryo, a foetus and a newborn baby, for example. Furthermore, it is not our intention to proceed to genetic engineering, but to treat infertile couples.

The ethical point of excess embryos is a good one. The couple decide how many embryos they would wish to have transferred; one, two or three, and the exact number of ripe eggs fertilized to fulfil this. The only source of excess embryos would be transfer difficulties or failures when the embryo(s) would be best frozen and transferred at a more favourable time. The slight success of the method has been dependent upon the production of two embryos, as this increases the chance of a successful pregnancy. Because there are both failed fertilizations and embryo cleavage, we have previously fertilized as many ripe eggs as are available.

Human Life of Embryo is Common Sense

William Daniel

In his reply to various critics, Professor Carl Wood (4/5) reproaches me for trying to impose on others the 'Roman Catholic teaching that a two-cell embryo, which cannot be seen by the naked eye, is human life', and yet he himself had earlier assured us that 'the utmost respect for human life pervades the whole in vitro programme'.

One sees the same kind of inconsistency in Robert Edwards (with Steptoe the co-developer of the first successful in vitro programme). On the one hand he mocked at those who regarded fertilization 'as a kind of holy event above the interference of man', and yet recalled: 'We were also aware that our work would enable us to examine a microscopic human being — one in its very earliest stages of development.'

That the life of the embryo is human life is not a Roman Catholic dogma. It is a common sense philosophical conclusion based on the biological facts. The embryo has life; it is a human embryo, and therefore the life it has is human — not that of some other species.

The phrase behind which Professor Wood shelters, 'potential human life', makes no sense to me. Certainly, the embryo is only a potential baby, just as a baby is only a potential adult. Yet the life whose evidence we see with the naked eye in baby and adult is human life. Why should we deny this attribute to the life of the microscopic embryo, when the biological continuity between all three is total and unbroken? My life began when my mother conceived me.

There is a strange contradiction in his last paragraph which should not be allowed to pass uncommemorated. On the one hand he says that the parents are consulted as to how many embryos they would wish to have transferred, 'and the exact number of ripe eggs (are) fertilized to fulfil this'. I for one would have welcomed this news. But at the end he says: 'Because there are both failed fertilizations and embryo cleavage, we have previously fertilized as many ripe eggs as are available.' If his tenses mean anything he is referring to present practice. Which are we to believe?

In his original letter (18/4), where he said that 'the whole point of freezing embryos is to preserve life, not destroy it', I wish he could have found space for some of the reservations he expressed in an interview on the ABC 'Science Show' a fortnight earlier: 'We don't even know that it is possible yet. Alan (Trounson) is reasonably confident, but it's not possible in all species to do this freezing and thawing. The early studies do show that it may be possible. That is about as far as we could go at the moment.' So I suppose the experiments will 'respectfully' continue.

5 The Moral Status of the Embryo: Two viewpoints

Brian Johnstone

In this chapter I understand 'moral status' as responding to the questions: how should we regard the gametes (the egg and sperm cells before fertilization) and the embryo and how should we behave towards them? These are, of course, much debated issues. I propose to deal with them only insofar as they are relevant to IVF and ET. I do not intend to attempt to consider all the moral issues raised by this procedure.

In discussions on these matters frequent use is made of such expressions as 'potential human life', 'potential human being', and 'potential person'. As a first step I will clarify this difficult notion 'potential'. The word is used in at least three ways.

Potential in the 'Weak' Sense

In this sense of the word one thing is said to have the 'potential' to become another if it could be transformed into the other by any kind of cause. It has been argued that an embryo has a potential to become a human being only in this weak sense.[1] Those who consider the embryo only a 'weakly' potential human being do not regard it as a human being or require that it be respected as such.

Potential in the 'Strong' Sense

Others would challenge the use of 'potential' in the weak sense when applied to the embryo. The embryo, after all, is not 'turned into' a human being by some purely extrinsic cause; it has a capacity for development within itself. Thus, they would speak of the embryo as 'fully potent for self-initiated development into a mature human being, if circumstances are co-operative'.[2] Edward A. Langerak has explained the difference in this way: a potential person is a being, not yet a person, that will become an actual person in the normal course of its development (e.g. a human foetus). A possible person is a being that could, under certain causally possible conditions, become an actual person (e.g. a human sperm or egg).[3] Potential in the weak sense would be better expressed as 'possibility'.

Some understand 'potential' in the strong sense to mean that all the higher stages of human development are present *in potentia* in the lower stages. Thus, the character of the foetus as potentially human raises it above the level of 'mere tissue'; it therefore evokes within us a sense of responsibility for its welfare. But it has less rights than it would have if it were fully born.[4] Others again hold for a successive actualization of the potential, so that one stage of development follows on another. The value of the potential and future state endows an object with value, but not the actual value of the future state. Thus the embryo has value, but not the same value as a person.[5]

Arguments from potential in the strong sense lead to limited moral conclusions: we should give the embryo respect but not necessarily the same respect we should give a mature human being.

Potential in the 'Statistical' Sense

There is a high probability that once the conceptus is formed, the new being will develop (one estimate is four out of five). In this sense, it could be said to have a 'potential' for development. Some would argue that we should not frustrate this potential.[6]

The moral implications of these facts, however, are not immediately clear. For example, if I act so as to prevent a particular embryo from developing into a mature human being, I have prevented it from achieving its 'potential'. But I may act so as to enable another embryo to come into being and develop *its* potential. If the desired result is achived, namely, the birth of a child, why should there be moral concern about the embryo, the potential of which was not actualized?[7] We are forced back to the question of whether there is something about each embryo which establishes its intrinsic value, independently of any actual development, and independently of the desires of other parties who may be involved. On this point opinions sharply divide.

How could we best express the condition of the embryo? It is *actually* living: it metabolizes, respires, responds to changes in the environment, grows and divides.[8] It is *actually* human; it pertains to the species *homo sapiens*. It is inappropriate, therefore, to refer to it as 'potential human life'. We could, however, say it is potentially a mature human being.

The Embryo

The embryo can develop into a mature human being. Harm wrought upon the embryo can result in harm to the mature human being. Since the degree of risk is unknown, some have argued that the procedure of IVF and ET constitutes unethical experimentation.[9] Others would propose that, provided the level of risk is approximately the same as that involved in the normal process of fertilization and gestation, the procedure could be acceptable.[10] This very serious question calls for attention whatever views may be held on the status of the embryo as such. The second opinion would seem to set a reasonable minimum. But a detailed discussion of this point would take us too far afield.

In dealing with the moral status of the embryo, I propose to use the more general term 'respect' rather than 'rights'. This will be sufficient for the purposes of the chapter.

One approach to the question can be outlined in a very simple and direct fashion. We accord respect to a person. But any line we attempt to draw, marking off a sharp distinction between embryo and person, appears to be arbitrary. Moral judgements should not be based on arbitrary distinctions. Therefore, we ought to regard the embryo as a person. This is clear as far as it goes. Both those who accept this argument and those who reject it, however, call on scientific evidence concerning the structure and development of the embryo to support their respective cases.

It is frequently unclear whether the arguments being proposed are arguments about the nature of the embryo, seeking to prove or disprove that it is a person, that is, a special kind of being; or arguments about the moral status of the embryo, seeking to prove or disprove that it ought to be regarded as a person, that is, the subject of respect. R. M. Hare has proposed that it is no use looking more closely at the embryo to satisfy ourselves whether it is really a person. The data we discover cannot provide a clear answer since the concept 'person' has fuzzy edges.[11]

One way of avoiding some of the confusion would be to use

'person' as a moral term to designate a subject of respect, and to use another concept as a descriptive term for the entity at a particular stage of development. Thus, we could say, the embryo will, unless something untoward happens, develop (at some stage) into a mature human being.

We accept a mature human being as a person. But we do so because we have *moral* reasons. For example, I may argue, this is a mature human being like myself. Therefore, I ought to accord him or her respect, just as I would want others to accord me respect. An embryo is clearly not a mature human being; it is conceivable, however, that we could have moral reasons for considering the embryo a person. The moral reasons which require us to accept a mature human being as a person will be applicable also to the embryo, depending on the continuity between the mature human being and the embryo.

The greatly increased scientific information about the processes of fertilization and embryonic development provides much evidence for the biological continuity between the embryo and the mature human being. On this basis, some of the more fanciful science fiction arguments proposed by some philosophers could be challenged.[12] There remains, however, the further question of how we are to interpret this biological data to decide which features are morally relevant and which are not. At this point fundamental philosophical differences enter into the arguments.

Joseph Fletcher, for example, would recognize birth as the moral marker for personhood.[13] Others would not recognize birth alone as definitive, but would consider also such factors as the capacity to envisage a future, desire to go on living, and autonomy.[14] Others again, would consider as morally relevant to personhood the very earliest developments in the life of the embryo.

A well-known case of this kind is presented by Paul Ramsey:

The human individual comes into existence first as a minute informational speck . . . (with the single exception of identical twins) no one else in the entire history of the human race has ever had or will ever have exactly the same genotype. Thus, it can be said that the individual is whoever he is going to become from the moment of impregnation. Thereafter, his subsequent development may be described as a process of becoming the one he already is.[15]

There are two key points in this argument: continuity of genetic constitution, and continuity of the individual. I propose that we examine these in turn.

Genetic Constitution

When sperm and egg unite this creates a distinct genetic entity. The genes of the later cells are not merely the product of mechanical division. The cells which develop later are different cells with their genetic composition produced by the self-replicating power of the original genotype. There is more involved here than the continuity between a blueprint and the completed house. There is an autonomous 'biological dynamic' from the beginning.[16]

It is not yet clear, however, whether, in dealing with the embryo in its early stages, we are dealing with a process through which the individual human being comes to be, or whether we are dealing already with the individual human being. Can we speak of a continuity of the individual from the earliest stages through to the mature human being?

Individuality

Self-identity in material, living things is not manifested by any part or parts which remain statically unchangeable and unchanged. Rather, it is manifested in an inner force which orders, governs, and integrates the unceasing interchange which is biological life. This would seem to allow for a gradual attainment of individuality within the continuing process of development. There is, furthermore, some 'hard data' which would tend to reinforce such a conclusion.

Some would maintain that, since twinning and recombination are possible in the early days after fertilization, irreversible individuality has not been achieved at this stage.[17] Ramsey would agree that these possibilities show the uncertainty of human individuation at conception.[18] If the uncertainty remains as long as twinning is possible, it would seem that individuality can be certainly established only at blastocyst stage (an embryo four to six days after fertilization). Before this period, the embryo may be considered as 'only potentially a human being'. This would imply that it is worthy of respect but not the same degree of respect as accorded to a mature human being. Noonan, on the other hand, points out that the probability of twinning or recombination occurring is very small. Thus, he argues, we should regard every embryo as if it were an individual.[19]

A 'Soul'

Those who argue for the existence of a 'soul' do not think of it as some kind of appended spiritual substance. Rather, 'soul' means something like 'dynamic principle of organization and development'. An ancient philosophical and theological tradition held for successive ensoulment of the embryo.[20] Fundamentally, this was an attempt to account for the different levels of organization which are evident in the process of development. Accordingly, it was proposed that in the early stages there was a 'vegetative' principle of organization, later an 'animal' principle, and later again a 'rational (human) soul'. In recent times some have taken up a version of this theory, leaving aside, of course, the inadequate biology.[21] A major difficulty, however, remains: how can we know with certainty when the rational, human soul is present?[22]

Roman Catholic theology has held that the human soul is present from the moment of conception ('immediate animation'). Some theologians now consider this doctrine uncertain and open to positive doubt.[23] Some of the reasons are the possibility of twinning and recombination and the loss of a large number of zygotes. If it is uncertain whether an individual is present, it must be uncertain whether an individual soul is present, and it seems anomalous that so many souls come into existence only to pass out of existence so soon.

The official Roman Catholic teaching on abortion does not depend upon the doctrine of 'immediate animation'. The relevant document stated clearly that it leaves undecided the question of the moment when the soul is 'infused'. The document makes two points: even if it is assumed that animation comes at a later point, the life of the foetus is 'incipiently human' as the biological sciences make clear; if the infusion of the soul at conception is at least probable, and the document claims that we will never establish the contrary with certainty, to take the life of the foetus is to run the risk of killing a human being.[24] The doctrine, then, is founded on probability. Some have set out to give a more detailed account of this kind of argument.

Probability

Once the conceptus is formed, the chances are four out of five that the new being will develop. (Different estimates are given, but the precise figures are not essential to the argument.) If I were to shoot at a movement in the bushes where there was a four out of five chance that the movement was that of a human being, I would be held blameworthy for taking such a high risk of injuring a human being. Similarly, if I act in a destructive way towards an embryo, where there is a four out of five chance that it will develop, I would be held blameworthy for taking such a high risk of destroying a human being.[25]

The criticism frequently levelled against this argument is as follows. The four out of five chance is the chance that this embryo *will later become* a person; the four out of five chance is not the chance that this *already is* a person.[26] My destructive act touches an entity which will probably *become* a person, not an entity which probably already *is* a person.

There is some confusion here because of the ambiguity of the word 'person'. The critics appear to take 'person' to mean the entity which emerges at the term of the process of development. I have suggested that we call this a 'mature human being'. Noonan clearly does not claim that there is a four out of five chance that the embryo (zygote) is already a mature human being. Obviously it is not. What he seems to be arguing is this. We know that four out of five embryos (zygotes) will develop into mature human beings. We do not know whether this particular embryo (zygote) will develop or not. But, unless there is evidence of damage, we must assume that there is a high probability that it will develop. That is, Noonan is seeking to establish that there is a probable continuity between this embryo (zygote) and a mature human being. Since we accord respect to the mature human being, we should accord the same respect to the embryo (zygote).

But why should we give the *same* respect, rather than a degree of respect corresponding to the degree of development? Noonan would reply: we are not justified in discriminating against a human life merely because of a difference in the realization of its potential.[27]

Those who argue for the personhood of the embryo from conception ultimately rest their case on two main points: an argument from probability, and the rejection of any dividing line between zygote and mature human being as arbitrary discrimination. The Lutheran theologian, Helmut Thielecke, would see the issue in relation to the real parenthood which the couple assume once impregnation takes place.[28]

The intentions of the participants and the objective design of the procedure are both directed to overcoming the arbitrary fate of infertility and to enabling a couple to meet their child as a person and, in so doing, to find their fulfilment as life-engendering persons. There is an implicit bias towards concern for life and for persons in the conduct of the procedure itself. I would argue that there is an inconsistency in re-introducing a new kind of arbitrariness in allowing excess embryos to be brought into being which cannot be implanted and which must be disposed of. (Some embryos, of course, are defective, so that even if they were implanted, there would be no prospect of development. I am concerned here only with those who do have such a prospect.) This arbitrariness touches the fate of beings which are living and human.

There are serious reasons for according these beings respect of a personal quality. There is no clear conflict with the respect due to other persons. Therefore, that respect should prevail and shape our behaviour towards these beings.

The creation of excess embryos and their consequent, inevitable destruction is discordant with such respect.

It may be possible, however. to eliminate this particular difficulty, for example, by preserving the gametes by freezing, thawing, and fertilizing at a time most suitable for successful implantation. If this can be done, there need be no excess, unimplanted embryos. This would remove one major moral objection to the procedure.

Others have begun work on the moral analysis of other features and wider implications.[29]

Unless something untoward happens, the embryo (zygote) will develop into a mature human being. With the possible exception of parthenogenesis, the gametes will not develop in this way. There is a special kind of continuity between embryo (zygote) and mature human being. It seems reasonable, then, to attribute to the embryo a moral significance which the gametes do not have. Even those who accord a fully personal respect to the embryo find no warrant for giving a similar respect to the gametes. That does not mean, however, that they have no moral significance at all. They are valuable to the couple as the possible precursors of the child they desire. In a sense, they are extensions of the prospective parents and should be dealt with according to their informed consent.

Helga Kuhse and *Peter Singer*

A living human embryo comes into existence as soon as a human egg and sperm have joined together. If the embryo is then implanted into the mother, it cannot be objected that the embryo has been denied any respect that might be due to it, for it has been placed into the environment that gives it the greatest possible chance of survival. But what if more eggs have been fertilized than can be re-implanted? What is to be done with them? Should they be frozen? But what if the couple who provided the egg and sperm do not wish to have the excess embryos re-implanted into the woman? (Perhaps the first embryo developed successfully, and they do not want any more children.) And what if, while not wishing to use the embryo themselves, the couple also do not like the idea of their genetic material being used by another couple? Should the embryos then be kept frozen for ever? What point would there be in that? Or can these excess embryos simply be tipped down the sink?

Many people find such questions bewildering. Seeing no way of answering them, they throw up their hands and say, 'It's all up to the individual's subjective judgement.' Our aim is to show that there is a rational answer to these questions, which should carry conviction with everyone who accepts one very widely held premise: that it is not wrong to destroy either the egg or the sperm before they have united.

On the basis of this premise we shall argue that there is no moral obligation to preserve the life of the embryo. Our argument applies specifically to the very early kind of embryo produced by the IVF programme. In other words, we are talking about an embryo that has developed for only some hours or at the most a day or two. It will only have divided a few times, into two, four, eight, or sixteen cells. (Technically, this is known as a zygote, but we shall continue to refer to it by the more widely known term 'embryo'.) At this stage, of course, the embryo has no brain, or even a nervous system. (Even the brain of a tadpole has more than 5000 cells.) The embryo could not possibly feel anything or be conscious in any way. Therefore, what we shall argue about this kind of embryo has no *necessary* application to an embryo at a later stage of development, for example, at a stage of development at which it does have a brain, and could feel pain.

The Premise

Our argument begins from the premise that it is not wrong to destroy either the egg or the sperm — the gametes, as they are collectively known — before they have united. We do not know of anyone who seriously asserts that the moral status of the egg and sperm before fertilization is such that it is wrong to destroy them. For instance, if a man is asked to produce a specimen of semen so that it can be tested to see if he is fertile, no one objects to the semen being tipped out once the test is complete. And after all, in our normal lives eggs and sperm are constantly being wasted. Every normal female between puberty and menopause wastes an egg each month that she does not become pregnant; and after puberty every normal male wastes millions of sperm in sexual intercourse in which contraceptives are used, or in which the woman is not fertile; and the same applies when he masturbates or has a nocturnal emission. Does anyone regard all of this as a terrible tragedy? Not to our knowledge; and so we do not think the premise of our argument is likely to be challenged.

We shall consider some imaginary stories. They do not describe any actual occurrences or even probable ones. We are using them to illustrate a moral point.

First Story

Doctors working on an IVF programme have obtained a fertile egg from a patient and some semen from the patient's husband. They are just about to drop the semen into the glass dish containing the egg, when the doctor in charge of the patient calls to say that he has discovered that she has a medical condition which makes pregnancy impossible. The egg could be fertilized and returned to the womb, but implantation would not occur. The embryo would die and be expelled during the woman's next monthly cycle. There is therefore no point in proceeding to fertilize the egg. So the egg and semen are tipped, separately, down the sink.

In accordance with our premise, as far as the moral status of the egg or the sperm before they have united is concerned, nothing wrong has been done.

Second Story

Everything happens exactly as in the first story, except that the doctor in charge of the patient calls with the bad news just *after* the egg and sperm have been placed in the glass dish and fertilization has already taken place. The couple are asked if they are prepared to consent to the newly created embryo being frozen to be implanted into someone else, but they are adamant that they do not want their genetic material to become someone else's child. Nor is there any prospect of the woman's condition ever changing, so there is no point in freezing the embryo in the hope of re-implanting it in her at a later date. The couple ask that the embryo be disposed of as soon as possible.

If the embryo has a special moral status that makes it wrong to destroy it, it would be wrong to comply with the couple's request. What, then, *should* be done with the embryo?

How plausible is the belief that it was not wrong to dispose of the egg and sperm separately but would be wrong to dispose of them after they have united? For those who believe that there is a real distinction between the two stories, here is a third story, not to be taken too seriously, but intended to bring out the peculiarity of that belief.

Third Story
This story begins just as the first one does. The doctor's call comes before the egg and sperm have been united, and so they are tipped, separately, down the sink. But as luck would have it, the sink is blocked by a surgical dressing. As a result, the egg has not actually gone down the drainpipe before the semen is thrown on top of it. A nurse is about to clear the blockage and flush them both away when a thought occurs to her: perhaps the egg has been fertilized by the semen that was thrown on top of it! If that has happened, or if there is even a significant chance of that having happened, those who believe that the embryo has a special moral status which makes it wrong to destroy it must now believe that it would be wrong to clear the blockage; instead the egg must now be rescued from the sink, checked to see if fertilization has occurred, and if it has, efforts should presumably be made to keep it alive.

On what grounds could one try to defend the view that the coming together of the egg and sperm makes such a crucial difference to the way in which they ought to be treated? We shall consider three possible grounds which have been put forward.

The Claim that a Human Life exists from Conception
The claim that a human life exists from the moment of conception is often used as an argument against abortion. We are not here

considering the issue of abortion but rather the moral status of the embryo. Nevertheless, the claim is relevant to our topic, because it is often assumed that once it is acknowledged that a human life exists from the moment of conception, it will also have to be conceded that from the moment of conception the embryo has the same basic right to life as normal human beings after birth.

To assess the claim that a human life exists from conception, it is necessary to distinguish two possible senses of the term 'human being'. One sense is strictly biological; a human being is a member of the species *homo sapiens*. The other is more restricted: a human being is a being possessing, at least at a minimal level, the capacities distinctive of our species which include consciousness, the ability to be aware of one's surroundings, to be able to relate to others, perhaps even rationality and self-consciousness.

When opponents of abortion say that the embryo is a living human being from conception onwards, all they can possibly mean is that the embryo is a living member of the species *homo sapiens*. This is all that can be established as a scientific fact. But is this also the sense in which every 'human being' has a right to life? We think not. To claim that every human being has a right to life solely because it is biologically a member of the species *homo sapiens* is to make species membership the basis of rights. This is as indefensible as making race membership the basis of rights. It is the form of prejudice one of us has elsewhere referred to as 'speciesism', a prejudice in favour of members of one's own species, simply because they are members of one's own species. The logic of this prejudice runs parallel to the logic of the racist who is prejudiced in favour of members of his race simply because they are members of his race.[30] If we are to attribute rights on morally defensible grounds, we must base them on some morally relevant characteristic of the beings to whom we attribute rights. Examples of such morally relevant characteristics would be consciousness, autonomy, rationality, and so on, but not race or species.

Hence, although it may be possible to claim with strict literal accuracy that a human life exists from conception, it is not possible to claim that a human life exists from conception in the sense of a being which possesses, even at the most minimal level, the capacities distinctive of most human beings. Yet it is on the possession of these capacities that the attribution of a right to life, or of any other special moral status, must be based.

The Claim from the Potential of the Embryo

It may be admitted that the embryo consisting of no more than sixteen cells cannot be said to be entitled to any special moral status because of any characteristics it actually possesses. It is, once again, far inferior to a tadpole in respect of all characteristics that could be regarded as morally relevant. But what of its potential? Unlike a tadpole, it has the potential to develop into a normal human being, with a high degree of rationality, self-consciousness, autonomy, and so on. Can this potential justify the belief that the embryo is entitled to a special moral status?

We believe it cannot, for the following reason. Everything that can be said about the potential of the embryo can also be said about the potential of the egg and sperm. The egg and sperm, if united, also have the potential to develop into a normal human being, with a high degree of rationality, self-consciousness, autonomy, and so on. On the basis of our premise that the egg and sperm separately have no special moral status, it seems impossible to use the potential of the embryo as a ground for giving it special moral status.

It is, of course, true that something may go wrong. The egg may be surrounded by semen, and yet not be fertilized. But it is also true that something may go wrong with the development of the embryo. It may fail to implant. It may implant but spontaneously abort. And so on. There is a possibility of something going wrong at every stage, from the production of egg and sperm right through to the time at which there is a rational and self-conscious being. That there is one more stage that the egg and sperm must go through, compared to the embryo, can scarcely make a decisive difference.

The Uniqueness of the Embryo

Some will concede that there is a sense in which both the embryo and the egg and sperm, taken separately, have the same potential, namely the potential to develop into a mature human being. Yet, they will want to say, there is a difference between these two forms of potential. As long as the egg and sperm are separate, the genetic nature of the individual human being that may come to exist is still to be determined. We have no way of telling which of the hundreds of thousands of sperm in a drop of semen will fertilize the egg. The unique genetic constitution of the embryo, on the other hand, has been determined for all time.

Can this difference provide a reason for giving the embryo higher status than the egg and sperm? Surely not, for the difference still does not show that the embryo has a different potential from the egg and sperm. The egg and sperm has the potential to develop into a mature human being. There are no genetically indeterminate human beings, and every genetically determinate human being is unique, with the exception of identical twins, triplets, and so on. Thus, the uniqueness of the embryo is nothing *additional* to its potential for becoming human. Why should our inability to tell which sperm will fertilize the egg make such a difference? If we were better able to predict which sperm would fertilize the egg, would we then say that the egg and sperm were now entitled to the same moral status as the embryo?

If it is uniqueness as such that we are talking about, and not the potential to develop into a mature human being, we should also remember that it is not only human beings who are genetically unique. Each individual chimpanzee is genetically unique too; so is each individual pig, and each individual rat, and each individual sparrow. Does that entitle them to special moral status? (Is it less evil to kill one of a pair of identical twins than it is to kill one of a pair of fraternal twins?)

Finally, if uniqueness is thought to be a basis for special moral status, what will happen when advances in the technique of cloning make it possible for each human cell to become an embryo? An embryo that is developed from the nucleus of a human cell in this manner would not be unique. Any other embryo developed in the same manner from a cell taken from the same person would be genetically identical to it. Would this mean that a cloned embryo would not have the moral status of a normal embryo? This seems an absurd conclusion; certainly it is one that cuts against all the other arguments we have been considering, for a cloned embryo is as much a living human being, and as much a potentially rational and self-conscious being, as a normal embryo.

Since none of these three grounds suffice to support a sharp distinction between the moral status of the embryo and that of the egg and sperm, we are left with just three possibilities: we must find another plausible reason for making this distinction, or we must abandon our initial premise, which was that the egg and sperm are not entitled to a special moral status which would make it wrong to destroy them, or we must hold that the embryo in its very earliest stage of life is also not entitled to a special moral status which would make it wrong to destroy it. We can find no other plausible reason for making the distinction. Our premise still seems well grounded. Hence we conclude that the newly created embryo is not entitled to a special moral status which makes it wrong to destroy it.

Our conclusion is contrary to the views of many theologians, including those of Dr Brian Johnstone which are set out in the first part of this chapter. On the other hand it does not seem to be at odds with the views of our community as a whole. There appears to be little or no opposition to the use of intrauterine devices, or IUDs, as a means of preventing pregnancy. There is evidence that these devices often work not strictly as contraceptives, that is, not by preventing conception but by ensuring that any egg that is fertilized will fail to implant in the womb. The fertilized egg, or embryo, is then expelled from the womb and dies. If the embryo, from its earliest stages, were entitled to a special moral status which makes it wrong to kill it, the use of IUDs would be a serious violation of that special moral status.

We are not claiming that two wrongs make a right. We have argued that the embryo in its earliest stages does not have a special moral status that makes it wrong to kill it. Hence we do not think that it is wrong to use an IUD, or to discard any excess embryos produced by IVF techniques. We have mentioned IUDs only to make the point that anyone who objects to the disposal of excess embryos produced in the course of attempts at IVF should also, to be consistent, object just as strongly to the use of an IUD. Anyone who calls for a ban on the use of IVF because it may lead to the discarding of human embryos will be on very weak ground unless he or she also calls for a ban on the use of IUDs.

The view we have argued for justifies the common sense reaction which we believe most readers will have had to the three stories we told earlier. If you felt that it would be absurd to hold that the medical staff are under a moral obligation to try to rescue the egg that may have been accidentally fertilized in the blocked sink, you were right. Similarly, whether the doctor's call came a minute before the egg and sperm were to be united, or a minute afterwards, makes no crucial difference. In none of these cases has a being come into existence which is capable of feeling or experiencing anything at all. In none of these cases is there a being that has a right to life.

6 Informed Consent by Participants: Who participates? Who consents?

B. E. Carey

Informed consent is one of the most commonly mentioned difficulties in human experimentation because, by definition, the word 'informed' implies complete knowledge, while in experimentation or research, the anticipated result is the acquisition of knowledge. Hence the difficulty in determining what constitutes both 'informed' and 'consent'. Most challenges to the authority for experimentation usually centre on the nature of consent, and the right to make such consent. Free, informed consent is crucial to participants in the IVF and ET programme. Before the matter of consent is considered, the question should be asked 'who participates', in terms of who has to give consent and, how is such consent to be given?

Who Participates?

The important relationship between researcher and participant is often highlighted in medical research, as the experimentation deals not with the abstract but with human beings and potential human beings. Guttentag[1] speaks of the relationship between researcher and subject in this way: 'In experimentation on human beings, experimenter and the experimental subject are fellow human beings; the veterinarian and his animal, the engineer and his machine are not.' This may sound very simple, but it is profoundly important. For, out of such awareness comes respect for the human subject and, in IVF research, that additional respect for the embryo which is an integral part of the relationship between researcher and participants.

Normally the participants in IVF research would be a married couple, from whom the eggs and sperm would be obtained. There are other options, however, which are presently outside the guidelines adopted by the Queen Victoria Medical Centre: eggs from the wife could be fertilized by donor sperm and transferred to the wife's uterus or to that of another woman; the husband's sperm could be used to fertilize donor eggs which could be transferred to his wife's uterus or to the uterus of the egg donor or another woman; donor eggs could be fertilized with donor sperm and then transferred to the wife's uterus or to that of the egg donor or another woman; or the wife could donate eggs and the husband sperm so that any resulting embryo could be transferred to the uterine cavity of another woman.

As the role of the participants varies in these situations, it raises the question of just who gives consent. To take this a step further, if the egg is donated, should the woman who donates the egg give the necessary consent for the action taken with the egg and later the embryo, or should the future recipient of the embryo give consent? Although there is a similarity here between adopting an egg or embryo and adopting a child in that the egg or embryo has the potential to become a child, this issue still needs to be resolved if and when donor eggs are used. The proposed changes in parliamentary legislation on the status of children conceived as a result of AID and ET may cover some of the problems raised.

The Nature of Consent

The core principle of medical ethics is that of free and informed consent, arising out of the Nuremberg Code (1946–49):

The voluntary consent of the human subject is absolutely essential. This means that the person involved should have legal capacity to give consent; should be so situated as to be able to exercise free power of choice, without the intervention of any element of force, fraud, deceit, duress, overreaching, or other ulterior form of constraint or coercion; and should have sufficient knowledge and comprehension of the elements of the subject matter involved as to enable him to make an understanding and enlightened decision. This latter element requires that before the acceptance of an affirmative decision by the experimental subject there should be made known to him the nature, duration and purpose of the experiment; the method and means by which it is to be conducted; all inconveniences and hazards reasonably to be expected; and the effects upon his health or person which may possibly come from his participation in the experiment.[2]

Further declarations such as that of Helsinki (1964) have reaffirmed the Nuremberg Code, adding to the matter of consent and obligation of the researcher the freedom of the subject to withdraw from the experiment at any time. Under the third section of the Helsinki declaration on non-therapeutic clinical research it says:

Clinical research on a human being cannot be undertaken without his free consent after he has been fully informed; if he is legally incompetent, the consent of the legal guardian should be procured.

The subject of clinical research should be in such a mental, physical and legal state as to be able to exercise fully his power of choice.

Consent should, as a rule, be obtained in writing. However, the responsibility for clinical research always remains with the research worker; it never falls to the subject, even after consent is obtained.

The investigator must respect the right of each individual to safeguard his personal integrity, especially if the subject is in a dependent relationship to the investigator.

At any time during the course of clinical research the subject or his guardian should be free to withdraw permission for research to be continued. The investigator or the investigating team should discontinue the research if in his or their judgement it may, if continued, be harmful to the individual.[3]

These two significant declarations form the substance and background for any discussion on the nature of consent, but what constitutes informed consent? What kind of information and what manner of informing fulfils the duty of the researcher towards his or her subject? This issue is often complex. How much information constitutes a reasonable explanation of procedures and expectations? Can the necessary information concerning the proposed research be explained in non-technical language that can be understood in a way that does not place 'unreal' expectations on the proposed research programme? Consent in this sense is not purely a legal matter but raises the hopes and fears of the subject in a far more objective way in terms of the success and risks of the experiment. Informed consent focusses closely on the essential aspects of knowing, because implied in knowledge is the dimension of failure and risk as well as hope for success.

Christian medical ethics emphasize responsibility and freedom of the subject and researcher, enabling the subject to be fully aware of that to which he is consenting. Any violation of human rights raises the fact that moral progress has been denied. This progress is not an end product as emphasized by Pappworth: 'An experiment is ethical or not at its inception, and does not become so *post hoc* because it achieved some measure of success.'[4] Informed consent freely given and able to be freely withdrawn is essential to a Christian ethical viewpoint. This viewpoint is no different from other ethical ones based on medical declarations, or on other ethical methodologies.

Consenting for Whom?

With IVF and ET, the adult participants in the research programme have given their consent to the initial action of collecting eggs and sperm. Their consent, however, is not centred on themselves but 'another'. May argues:

Since every human being is of incomparable worth, with inherent dignity and value that transcend the society in which he or she lives, each human being has the right to be regarded as one who cannot rightfully be subordinated to that society or to any person within it.[5]

For May, the egg and sperm which go to constituting the embryo are subjected to the will of others and therefore this is contrary to the right of being a human. He argues further that IVF research is non-therapeutic, because it has no possible medical benefit to its subject, namely, the child-to-be; no disease is diagnosed, cured or prevented as a result of the procedure, and therefore there is really no patient. He continues by suggesting that as no consent is given by the embryo, the 'parents' are not entitled to take such action. May denies that enabling a couple to have a child by this method constitutes worth, and he strongly opposes IVF on a number of grounds, from the perspective of natural law, but in this instance on the grounds that an adult cannot give consent on behalf of the embryo-to-be. He further believes that proxy consent is wrong as it contravenes a right.

Paul Ramsey extends this argument even further to suggest that it is false to use the word 'consent' when referring to 'proxy consent' because in this situation there is no meaning to the concept of consent. The embryo has been created by the deliberate decision of adults and therefore no consent on its part was ever considered. Ramsey[6] further argues that experiments designed for the benefit of others (i.e. having a child) can constitute a 'wrong'. He writes:

To attempt to consent for a child to be made an experimental subject is to treat a child as not a child. It is to treat him as if he were an adult person who has consented to become a joint adventurer in the common cause of medical research. If the grounds for this are alleged to be the presumptive or implied consent of the child, this must simply be characterized as a violent and a false presumption. Non-therapeutic, non-diagnostic experimentation involving human subjects must be based on true consent if it is to proceed as a human enterprise. No child or adult incompetent can choose to become a participating member of medical undertakings, and no one else on earth should decide to subject these people to investigations having no relation to their own treatment. That is a canon of loyalty to them. This they claim of us simply by being a human child or incompetent. When he is grown, the child may put away childish things and become a true volunteer. This is the meaning of being a volunteer; that a man enter and establish a consensual relation to some joint venture for medical progress.[6]

Ramsey's argument is not to be construed that violence is being done to the human being on whose behalf consent is given, but rather to suggest that it is spurious to accept that consent has been received.

The argument over the ability to give consent for another is one of the many objections to IVF by moral theologians, especially those of the Catholic Church's tradition. Some Protestant theologians besides Ramsey agree with those objections; others hold more closely to the Helsinki declaration as an adequate basis on which consent can be given by adults in such experimentation as IVF.

The issue of the consent of the embryo may sound ludicrous, but it is precisely because consent cannot be given that the opposing moral argument is that the research should not be carried out.

This type of argument should also be presented for normal human reproduction. One does not hear opponents of IVF and ET asking the same questions about consent and risk involved in the normal process, and so I wonder when the last embryo was consulted or gave consent to its environment. Does the embryo generally have any status or rights?

The Rights of the Embryo and the Needs of the Prospective Parents

The right to procreate has been an assumed right of society generally, thereby implying the power of adults to give informed consent to research programmes designed to help with their infertility. One may argue that one is a complete human, male or female, without having to procreate to become complete, yet there are pressures and desires to have children. For some moral theologians, such as Paul Ramsey, IVF is wrong because it denies the rights of an embryonic human being, and moreover the damage that may be caused by this type of fertilization may not be observed for a few years. Ramsey writes:[7] 'In Vitro Fertilization constitutes unethical medical experimentation on possible future human beings and, therefore, is subject to absolute moral prohibition', and 'researchers cannot exclude the possibility that they will do irreparable damage to the child-to-be.'

Informed consent by the prospective parents relates not only to their right to procreate but also to their needs, namely to have a child. In the view of Fletcher and others human needs, in this case the need to have a child, have a higher priority than embryo rights:

Needs are the moral stabilizers, not rights. The legalistic temper gives first place to rights, but the humanistic temper puts needs in the driver's seat. If human rights conflict with human needs, let needs prevail. If medical care can use genetic controls preventively to protect people from disease or deformity, or to ameliorate such things, then let so-called 'rights' to be born step aside. If research with embryos and foetal tissue is needed to give us the means to cure and prevent the tragedies of 'unique genotypes', even though it involves the sacrifice of some conceptuses, then let rights take a back seat.[8]

Fletcher's argument goes further when he suggests that human values are related to needs and therefore we must consider the entire concept of consent and parenting in terms of what constitutes a human being and human reproduction. By consenting to IVF research, potential parents are embarking upon a planned parenthood:

It seems to me that laboratory reproduction is radically human compared to conception by ordinary heterosexual intercourse. It is willed, chosen, purposed and controlled, and surely these are among the traits that distinguish *homo sapiens* from others in the animal genus, from the primates down. Coital reproduction is, therefore, less human than laboratory reproduction — more fun, to be sure, but with our separation of babymaking from lovemaking, both become more human because they are matters of choice, and not chance. This is, of course, essentially the case for planned parenthood.[9]

Although the question of informed consent for the participant in IVF is clear in regard to the initial implantation of the embryo, the use of an excess of normal zygotes (embryos just after fertilization) for experimentation, and the monitoring of the implanted embryo raise further issues of consent. The ethical guidelines adopted by the Queen Victoria Medical Centre cover these and the following points from the guidelines are relevant:

As the entire procedure of IVF and ET involves a series of steps occurring over a variable period of time, it is important that the parents should be informed that their consent to IVF and ET is such that they can withdraw at any stage.

As a freezing technique has now been developed to allow the development of the zygote to be temporarily suspended by freezing, it is recommended that this technique be used when the IVF procedure has produced an excess of normal zygotes and/or the present conditions for implantation are less than optimal. It is anticipated that implantation will take place as soon as conditions are considered optimal. Should abnormal zygotes be detected, it is recommended that they should be appropriately examined to find out the cause of the abnormality and thereby, hopefully, enable it to be prevented in the future.

Parents will give informed consent to any procedure that may be undertaken on the zygote.

Once the embryo has been implanted, should any foetal abnormality be detected, before any action is taken, the parents should be fully informed of the nature of any foetal abnormality so that they can make a decision concerning termination or continuation of the pregnancy.[10]

Finally, the participants by giving informed consent are free to withdraw from the IVF research as they are also free to withdraw their zygotes. This freedom is crucial and central to the whole ethical aspect underlying the nature of consent.

In my opinion, human needs can be acknowledged as the overriding factor involved in the consent to IVF without diminishing respect for human life in its embryonic form.

7 Sexual Ethics in relation to IVF and ET: The fitting use of human reproductive power

William J. Daniel

I recall how once in my student days, when we were on holiday on the south coast of New South Wales, one of my fellow students went out for the day hitch-hiking. The driver who picked him up asked him how he earned his bread. 'Well actually', he replied, 'I'm a seminarian'. A moment's pause. 'Oh right!' came the reply. 'I know your place. It's just out of Berry on the highway.' The place referred to was the artificial breeding centre, where semen was prepared for the artificial insemination of dairy cows.

If the connection between artificial insemination of cattle and a seminary seems remote (however well founded etymologically), the connection between IVF and sexual ethics may seem no less remote, even to the thoughtful observer. Indeed, some would say that the seminarian story is particularly apt, that IVF is a triumph of veterinary science, and should have stopped there. Others would think that sexual ethics concern the way we relate to one another as sexed persons; whereas IVF belongs to the world of white coats and operating theatres. Whatever ethics are involved will be medical ethics, surely: concern for the welfare of the patient, informed consent, and so on.

In this connection it is worth noting that the question has been raised whether the procedure of IVF and ET is to be regarded as properly a medical procedure at all. R. G. Edwards comments on the 'remarkable opinion' that this procedure is not a cure for infertility, that the woman's condition remains as it was before. He argues against this by analogy with the giving of insulin to correct diabetes, or the giving of spectacles to correct defective eyesight. 'In fact,

most medical treatment, particularly of constitutional or genetic disorders, is similarly symptomatic in nature. Exactly the same argument
applies to the cure of infertility: should patients have their desired
children, the treatment would have achieved its purpose. To state
the opposite is nonsense.'[1] There is a good, bluff common sense
about this reply, but the objection is not quite as nonsensical as he
maintains. Infertility is a special sort of disease: it is more a symptom
than a disease. What we recognize as disorder or impairment is the
blockage of the woman's Fallopian tubes. So it would be true therapy
to reconstruct her blocked tubes to enable her to conceive a child in
the normal way. What is being treated in the case of IVF, however,
is her desire to have a child,[2] by the introduction of biological technology into the marriage relationship and into the making of the
child. It is argued that 'to construe this procedure as a practice of
medicine we have to construe medicine to be devoted to the satisfaction of desires'.[3]

I mention this argument, not because I think it is an irrefutable
objection to the procedure, but because it does bring out the difficulty
of applying standard medical ethics to the question.

The healing function of medicine usually carries its own justification. Disease is an evil, and medicine sets out to fight it. Even if
the treatment causes harm in the process (e.g. the loss of function
in an amputation or the debilitating effects of some therapeutic drugs),
we can weigh the loss against the advantage of having the disease
cured or controlled.

But when medical or biological skill is turned from curing dys-
function to enhancing function, its justification is less simple and
obvious. It is one thing to give drugs to enable an arthritic patient
to walk; it is another to give drugs to an athlete to enable him to
break a record.

It is not wrong *per se* for the medical profession to go beyond the
curing of disease to the 'satisfaction of desires', but it must acknowledge that it is going beyond its basic therapeutic role, and
answer any questions that may be asked about the reasonableness
of the desires and the propriety of the means used.

I doubt if the most ardent advocate of zero population growth
would contest the general reasonableness of the desire of a childless
couple to have a child. Some would go further and urge their *right*
to have children, and imply a corresponding duty on the medical
profession to supply these children if the means are available.[4] I would

suggest a more modest reading of the United Nations Declaration of Human Rights, where it mentions 'the right to marry and found a family' (article 16). This surely implies a right *to be allowed* to marry and found a family — against racist marriage laws, for example, or forcible sterilization or coercive birth control programmes. But surely this does not constitute a claim on society to provide expensive technology to give me a family, any more than society is obliged to find me a mate.

On the other hand, some would dispute the reasonableness of the desire, blaming it on to a role stereotype of the woman. 'There were times when I was depressed', said one mother of an IVF baby, 'feeling that somehow you weren't a real woman unless you were fertile'. An extreme feminist might take umbrage at such a feeling, and claim that the cure for it is not IVF but a change in the attitudes of society. I doubt if the woman in question would be much helped by this approach. Her need is real enough to her, and the object of it, surely, is a good one: the having of a baby.

I propose that we accept that the desire of a childless couple to have a child of their own is a reasonable one. The ethical question then turns around the propriety of the means used. The question is whether it is a fitting use of the human reproductive power, of our sexuality.

There are questions of fittingness that cannot readily be resolved into a kind of moral profit and loss account of pleasure or pain or of any other kind of advantage or disadvantage. One can see this in the area of experimentation with human subjects (to take a medical example). It is not enough for an experimenter to have found subjects silly enough or desperate enough to undergo his experiments. It is recognized that there are experiments that may indeed produce an advance in knowledge but are so random or unnecessary or destructive that they should not be performed on a human subject, even with consent — and even if the subject were a criminal already condemned to death.

A utilitarian might agree, but argue that such experiments would be ultimately counterproductive in their brutalizing effects on the experimenters or on the profession. A more spontaneous and commonsense reaction, however, is that it is not necessary to calculate imagined consequences: it is enough to recognize that such experiments are an offence to human dignity. We should not use human subjects as we would (rightly or wrongly) use animals for experiments.

The quest for the fitting, for what is appropriate to the dignity of the human person, is nowhere more marked than in the area of sexual ethics.

This assertion would not be universally accepted. There is high and low in the area of sexual ethics as there is in churchmanship. Someone for whom sex is simply 'the healthiest and most important human sport', and for whom no form of sexual behaviour is worthy of censure 'unless it has demonstrable ill effects on the individual who practices it, or on others',[5] would regard the assertion as nonsense and this whole chapter as a waste of time.

But there are others who would ask how we are to identify ill effects if we have no idea of what constitutes human flourishing in this area. And they might ask further whether right and wrong is *primarily* a matter of ill effects at all. When I distort the truth there may or may not be ill effects from my lying, but the primary ill, which is not just an effect, is that I am behaving as a liar, am a liar.

The abuse of sexuality can indeed cause ill effects that are readily observable: heartbreak, fatherless children, disease. But even if such ills are avoided there is still a lack of fittingness. The absolutely discreet adulterer is still unfaithful. The most beneficient Don Juan is still a libertine.

The difficulty about out present topic is that sexual ethics generally deal with the relationship between sexed persons, one to one. In the case of IVF and ET, however, the relationship between man and woman is depersonalized, technologized. Is it any more personal than the relationship between a blood donor and the eventual recipient? Is it any more sexual than such a relationship? And so when we seek to set this procedure within the framework of sexual ethics, many of the usual reference points no longer apply.

The enterprise of sexual ethics is an attempt to provide guidance for the personalizing and socializing of the sexual instinct. It seeks to identify the *humanum*, what is fitting and ennobling in the sexual relationship; to stigmatize what it sees as unworthy or irresponsible conduct. It deals with attitudes, with their physical expression, with the begetting of children, and the continuing relationship of marriage or family. There are sufficient points of contact to enable IVF and ET to be called a question in sexual ethics, but it is apparent that it raises some quite special problems.

One useful reference point is the discussion of the morality of artificial insemination in the human (AIH or AID). Christian ethicists have taken strong exception to insemination from anonymous donors (AID) as being contrary to the covenant of marriage,[6] but even AIH has not gone without objection. In an address in 1951, Pope Pius XII argued that to consider intercourse of husband and wife as simply an expedient for the transmission of semen would be turning 'the family sanctuary' of marriage into 'a mere biological laboratory'.[7] The sexual act is a personal action, he argued, which expresses also the love and mutual self-giving of the partners.

One does not need to be a Roman Catholic to share this concern. Helmut Thielicke, the German Lutheran ethicist, says that the couple are created for each other as 'one flesh', and 'that *in* this oneness they are to satisfy the command "Be fruitful and multiply"'. The personal unity of man, wife and child would therefore be ruptured by any isolation of the biological act of procreation'.[8]

Leaving religious considerations aside, one can argue that there is something intrinsically valuable that our human beginnings are in a human act of love between our parents. Of course not all conceptions can lay claim to this dignity; nevertheless, as Paul Ramsey remarks, 'an ethics . . . that *in princple* sunders these two goods . . . pays disrespect to the nature of human parenthood'.[9] This touches on something that differentiates human procreation from the breeding of animals.

Ramsey's book, *Fabricated Man*, from which the above quotation was taken, deals mainly with the Brave New World projects and the dreams of certain geneticists. One can challenge the assumption of god-like wisdom that lies behind the projects for designing and engineering a better type of human being than the randomness of nature provides. But more fundamental is the objection that the depersonalizing of human procreation is an offence to our humanity. If we feel a repugnance for the selective breeding that the Nazis are said to have encouraged, it need not be because we dislike Aryans.

The procedure of IVF and ET is a prerequisite for genetic engineering, but it does not necessarily lead to it, and it deserves to be considered on its own merits. The procedure is depersonalized to the extent that it involves the participation of a medical technologist. But what he is trying to do is to achieve for the couple what their lovemaking is unable to do. He is not sundering human procreation from human love to make hatcheries for a Brave New World. This is not the sundering 'in principle' to which Ramsey rightly objected. It is no denial of the human link between love and procreation, but an attempt to achieve the procreation that their love seeks. It is true to the relationship of the couple, and in its way expresses it. As the woman previously quoted expressed it in a Melbourne newspaper interview: 'We have a total involvement with each other, and this baby is an expression of [my husband's] love for me and my love for him.'

It will be a matter for concern to some that the semen of the husband is obtained by masturbation. This would have been a much greater issue fifty years ago than it is today. Karl Menninger observes that from having been *the* sin of youth, masturbation has become almost overnight no sin at all. He finds this particularly significant of the changed temper, philosophy, and morality of the twentieth century, and links it to the general waning of the sense of sin, and its replacement by the notion of 'crime'; but this is a matter that lies outside our present topic.[10]

One's view of masturbation will vary according to one's general view of human sexuality. If one operates on a 'healthy sport' view of sexual activity, it may be regarded as an ever available source of good, clean fun. Some may even prefer it to other forms of sexual activity, as some card players may prefer patience to bridge. But if sexuality is seen in terms of human relationship, and sexual acts as an expression of a very special love, then masturbation must be viewed as something defective. If sexual acts are a communication, masturbation is a talking to oneself. If sexual acts are to have a meaning, masturbation is a nonsense.

But in the context of IVF, it may be argued that it does have a meaning and purpose, and that this is one of the meanings of our sexuality overall. It is not the act of one turned in on himself; it is, in the circumstances, an other-directed act.

Sexual ethics concerns the relationship between sexed persons. It is against human dignity to treat another person as an object, or as a mere instrument for the satisfaction of one's own desires. Sexuality offers the opportunity for a most intimate communication between persons and, as in all communication, honesty and personal integrity become an issue. Sexuality also offers the opportunity for bringing new life into existence.

The connection between love and procreation is not fortuitous. One could give a very good theological basis for it, but we need not go so far back. Leon Kass asks:

Is there possibly some wisdom in that mystery of nature which joins the pleasure of sex, the communication of love, and the desire for children in the very activity by which we continue the chain of human existence? Is biological parenthood a built-in 'device' selected to promote the adequate caring for posterity? Before we embark on new modes of reproduction, we should consider the meaning of the union between sex, love, and procreation, and the meaning and consequences of its cleavage.[11]

Kass is gloomy about IVF and ET, because he sees it as part of a process, which began with artificial insemination and will continue into genetic engineering, cloning, and the rest, resulting eventually in the destruction of *human* reproduction and the family, and exposing the future of the race to the same lack of wisdom that has led technological man to make such a mess of his material environment.

I believe he is being unduly pessimistic; that the procedure of IVF and ET does not inevitably lead to the subsequent horrors; that the justification of IVF simply to alleviate infertility in a married couple implies no logical justification for the further steps that would involve the mechanization of human reproduction or meddling with the genetic future of the race. But the word of warning should be heeded nevertheless.

By the development of modern methods of contraception, our generation has been fairly successful in separating the act of love from procreation. The achievement of IVF and ET has been to separate procreation from the act of love. I would have thought that no one in his right mind would have seen that as a positive value, but rather as a fairly desperate expedient to achieve for a couple what the act of love could not do for them.

I have argued that the desire of a childless couple to have a child is a reasonable one, and that the technological elements in IVF and ET are not so obtrusive as to depersonalize completely the procreation sought by the couple. It is not untrue to the relationship of the husband and wife, whose normal sexual expression is not enough to give them the child they desire.

We have been supposing all along that the procedure is to take place within the marriage situation. That limitation has been placed on the use of the procedure by the Melbourne team out of deference to the mores of society. It would be more reassuring if the limitation were imposed by them, and by those who fund their work, as a matter of principle rather than a matter of social expediency.

It would be idle for the medical technologists who have pioneered this procedure to say that it is not for them to dictate matters of right and wrong to society at large. They must assume responsibility for their own decisions and actions, and the more these touch at the roots of society — family and respect for human life — the greater their responsibility to see that their procedures should not undermine these foundations, however clamant the demands of those who come to them to have their desires satisfied.

The scope of this chapter has been very limited. It has had to ignore very important aspects of the question. I am not convinced, for example, that it is a responsible use of public money to spend so much to help so few when the health budget, as it affects the poor, is becoming more stringent. I am not satisfied that the procedure as currently practised is properly respectful of the human life of the embryo, with the process of multiple fertilization, selection, and the so far purely experimental freezing of the unused or unwanted embryos.

But as for what touches the area of human sexuality there are further adventures beckoning: surrogate mothers, host wombs, the artificial insemination of women who want a child but not a husband. I would share the view of the American commentators, Hellegers and McCormick: 'We see in these procedures grave assults on marriage and the family, to say nothing of the subtle devaluation of sexual intimacy that clings to them.'[12]

Instead of insisting on the right of a couple to have a child, as some have done, let us be mindful rather of the right of a child to have parents. And while we seek to satisfy the laudable desires of individuals let us not lose sight of the welfare of society at large, which depends so much on a right appreciation of marriage and of the dignity of human sexuality and procreation. That these are being subjected to such onslaughts today is no reason for adding a new onslaught from clinical technology.

8 IVF and the Human Family: Possible and likely consequences

John A. Henley

In 1979 the director of the Hastings Centre in New York, Dr Daniel Callahan, published a short article on 'the moral career of genetic engineering'.[1] Callahan pointed out that opponents of genetic engineering have based their arguments on moral principles but that, whatever the validity of these arguments may be, they have proven less than persuasive. The scientific community, legislators, and the general public seem to be more impressed by arguments which indicate the beneficial consequences of developing and applying new methods of human control over natural processes.

The new technique of IVF and ET seems to have generated an ethical debate which is taking the same course as that analysed by Callahan. At the time his article was published, one of the chief protagonists of a principled, as opposed to a consequentialist, approach to moral issues was arguing that it was not possible to test the new technique by morally permissible means because any attempt to do so involved some risk to a possible human being, the child-to-be.[2]

The joy of couples who, by means of the new technique, have recently become parents of infants who appear quite normal and healthy can scarcely be matched by the satisfaction of observers who judge the morality of human acts by their consequences, but the latter would appear to have been vindicated yet again. I suspect, however, that it would be premature for such a conclusion to be drawn. Not only do some of the consequences of the new technique remain to be seen, but their ethical implications require more attention than they tend to receive in the polarized debate between the upholders of moral principles and the consequentialists.

In this chapter, I propose to consider some of the possible, as well as more likely, consequences of IVF and ET for the family and society. In so doing, I shall not be content to indicate the beneficial or harmful aspects of such consequences but, where appropriate, I shall question the morality of the human situation brought about by the introduction of the new technique. In other words, just as I allow that divorce need not be morally wrong but nevertheless confirms that persons are not in a morally good situation, if not morally in the wrong, so I am prepared to concede that IVF and ET need not contravene any moral principle, but I am concerned to investigate whether this new technique places people in a situation that is morally less than satisfactory.

The Family

Since it seems reasonable to suggest that ethics must to some extent be concerned about human welfare, it can be stated at the outset that the new technique of IVF and ET is morally welcome because it enables some couples to bear the genetic offspring they desire. In view of the trouble to which they must go in order to achieve this desire, such couples might be expected to treat their children with especial love and care and, if so, this would be a consequence to be morally approved, provided, of course, that the family not turn in on itself to the detriment of all concerned. Beyond this, it can be added that any who regard marriage as incomplete if it fails to result in procreation could be expected to consider the new technique morally legitimate in so far as it helps in fulfilling this purpose. Such an expectation would appear to be strengthened by any disposition to prefer more, rather than less, children to be brought into the world. The Pastoral Constitution on the Church in the Modern World, issued by the Second Vatican Council, pronounces marriage and conjugal love to be 'by their nature ordained toward the begetting and educating of children' and describes children as 'the supreme gift of marriage' in view of the major contribution they make 'to the welfare of their parents'. The document also gives special praise to those couples 'who with wise and common deliberation, and with a gallant heart, undertake to bring up suitably even a relatively large family'.[3] Professor Peter Singer finds it puzzling that a group which would share this outlook on marriage has expressed opposition to the IVF programme in Melbourne since 'the whole aim of the programme is to create human life'.[4]

The scientific ground for IVF was prepared in the 1960s at a time when the Western world was experiencing what has been described as a 'revolution of rising expectations'. By offering the prospect of parenthood to couples who would otherwise remain childless, the new technique shows itself to be clearly a part of that revolution. In recent years, however, it has become apparent that there is a price to pay for any process of rapid growth, whether this price is financial, material, environmental or some other kind. Reason has been found to doubt whether the progress made, and the expectations that accompanied it, were unambiguously good. Similar doubts may arise concerning IVF because, however much the technique may be improved, it seems unlikely that all who participate in a programme are going to benefit by it. On the contrary, many who have conceived a new hope of becoming parents are going to suffer disappointment at best, bitterness at worst. In view of this problem and of its potential for further harm, participants in the Melbourne programme are invited to join support groups, in and through which they may be helped to cope with difficulties that may arise. Given that the programme is in operation, the establishment of these groups is morally responsible, but their necessity at least invites the question whether it was morally wise to embark upon the programme in the first place. It certainly seems doubtful whether the frustration caused to some couples can be justified by means of an analysis which simply weighs this cost against the benefit gained for others.

As far as the great value that some may attribute to the birth of children on theological or other grounds is concerned, it can be pointed out, of course, that such value may not be taken to justify every possible means of realizing it. As a means of procreation IVF may be rejected on the grounds not just of moral principle but also of expediency. It could be regarded as too expensive, for example. Instead of concentrating upon the means, however, I would prefer to raise a few questions about the ends, namely 'the begetting and educating of children'. For these may not be matters of unequivocal value. If we apply the famous 'open question' test of G. E. Moore and ask whether it is good for a couple to produce children and whether it is good for additional children to be born, the questions seem quite reasonable, which is not to suggest that in most cases they should be answered in the negative. They are reasonable questions because, as the Pastoral Constitution of the Second Vatican Council recognizes, marriage retains its value 'even when offspring are lacking — despite, rather often, the very intense desire of the couple'.[5] This indicates the possibility of being profoundly, but not indiscriminately, in favour of life and, if Professor Singer were less convinced of the 'fanaticism' of some who support a right to life and yet oppose IVF, he would be less puzzled by their opposition.

A programme of IVF does comprehend, however, that couples who seek to enter it may not all be pursuing what is good for them. For this reason it is necessary for applicants to be screened so that only those judged suitable will be admitted to the programme.[6] The grounds of such judgement are still being refined and are likely to vary from one institution to another, but a negative judgement may prove just as harmful to a couple as the disappointment that can attend admission to the programme. The necessity of screening, like that of support groups, seems to call the moral wisdom of the programme in question, especially when the intimate bearing of the required judgement is borne in mind. The judgement may be made largely on medical grounds relating to the health of the couple, especially the woman, but the question remains whether anybody possesses the insight and understanding to determine in advance that the claim of one couple to bear a child is inferior to that of another. It is one thing to point out that the vocation of a married couple need not include being parents; it is quite another to deny this aspect of the vocation to those who seek it.

Finally, as far as the family is concerned, something must be said about the child who becomes part of a family by means of IVF and ET. The apparent normality and health of the children so far born as a result of the new technique has already been noted and, in any event, it could seem hard to argue that they may encounter problems which could outweigh the good of their existence. For any problems presuppose the existence of a subject who experiences them, and they only appear as problems in the light of the hopes to which the birth of a child gives rise. The ontological priority of life over quality of life, however, does not entail an ethics of sheer fecundity, as I pointed out in connection with pronouncements made by the Second Vatican Council. Hence it is possible to envisage IVF and ET causing serious problems for children and families in such a way that the moral wisdom of the programme is again called in question. We shall have to wait and see, for example, whether or not the children produced by means of IVF and ET are disturbed by the knowledge of the special circumstances of their origin. If their sense of identity is disturbed, some will blame extraneous factors, such as the media for giving undue publicity to the novel arrivals, but it seems doubtful whether these will bear all the responsibility. The concern shown by some adopted children to find their natural parents has not been entirely a result of publicity given by the media.

It would appear, then, that the technique of IVF and ET offers some benefit to married couples but also brings actual and potential problems in its wake. In view of these problems, the value of a programme involving the new technique may, perhaps, be doubted. Does analysis of such a programme from a broader, social perspective yield a similar conclusion?

Human Society
The welfare of the family is clearly a matter of concern for society, which will have to assess, therefore, the likely consequences for the family of an IVF programme and their ethical implications. It should go without saying that evaluation of the costs and benefits of such a programme will need to include the human factor as well as the financial and material ones, which are more tangible. Beyond these fairly obvious points, however, there are further issues for society to face.

In the first place, attention will have to be given to the allocation of comparatively scarce and increasingly expensive medical resources. Some critics of modern medicine may argue that an IVF programme wastes these resources on a few privileged couples while poorer citizens still lack adequate medical attention. I think that this kind of argument can be dismissed on the grounds that it is economically naive and politically begs the question, and it also ignores the value to society of a creative medical service. Medical pioneers deserve the encouragement to implement new programmes and a fair opportunity to prove their worth so as to establish them. Another reason for this is the likelihood that the programme will generate additional knowledge of potential benefit to human beings and therefore to society. In the case of an IVF programme, a better understanding of the early stages of pregnancy may be anticipated and this contains the promise of future benefit to couples not involved in the programme and to their children. These considerations incline me to think that society could do well to make financial and material resources available to the programme at least for a stipulated time and also take steps to remove certain legal hindrances to it, in particular, the risk of claims for negligence against doctors or scientists involved in the programme. Having made this suggestion, however, I must immediately add some reservations about it.

It seems to me that society must reckon with the possibility that the establishment of an IVF programme will reduce public satisfaction with the medical service and do so on grounds which may not be set aside by any apparent success of the programme. Two reasons may be given for this, the first of which relates to a matter which is already of some public concern, namely, the frozen embryos that are a by-product of the programme and what is to be done with them.

Despite the puzzlement of Professor Singer, concern about the frozen embryos was bound to cause some opposition to the programme that is producing them. For, as he seems prepared to concede, destruction of these embryos could be regarded as equivalent to abortion, an issue which continues to trouble and divide society. Professor Singer points out that, apart from the programme, 'the embryos in question would never even have existed',[7] but the bearing of this statement on the moral and social issue is not clear. It is certainly not going to impress those whose concern about a right to life focusses on beings already in existence. In this connection, it may be noted, with some irony, that the very progress of biology and medicine in recent years would seem to have been a factor in an increased public awareness of the humanity of the embryo and the foetus. Although this does not prove that an embryo or foetus is a person with the same rights and privileges as other people, it does indicate that concern about the fate of the frozen embryos is likely to continue.

It is hardly an adequate response to this concern for a medical scientist to point out that a two-cell embryo 'cannot be seen by the naked eye'.[8] If it is judged to be human, which seems reasonable[9] and, still more, if it is to be regarded as a person, which is more debatable, then it enters into the arena of moral responsibility just as surely and to the same extent as other human beings or persons whom, for geographical or other reasons, the naked eye does not see. Indeed, since human beings made themselves more than usually responsible for its arrival on the scene, it can be argued that they have thereby become more responsible for its fate than they are with respect to others of their neighbours, near or far. Thus, concern about the frozen embryos not only calls public support for the IVF programme in question but casts further doubt upon its moral status.

An area of potential social concern is that IVF provides an additional means of separating 'lovemaking' from 'babymaking'. This may be taken to imply that the new technique is simply analogous to artificial insemination, which has not given rise to insurmountable problems.[10] I doubt whether the matter is as simple as this, however, because IVF does seem to go beyond artificial insemination in opening up possibilities of surrogate motherhood and genetic manipulation. It can, of course, be pointed out that these uses of the new technique and others, such as fertilization of women who may be single or homosexual, can be discouraged by appropriate legislation and regulations, but this may not be enough to satisfy those who are alarmed by the very possibility. Furthermore, there are movements afoot to extend the rights of single women and homosexuals and so any attempt to restrict their right to conceive a child is likely to produce a public debate which could be just as disturbing to society as that concerning abortion.

A society need not seek to avoid contentious issues at all costs but, in the context of my argument, the likelihood of public concern about possible uses of IVF and ET may be taken as yet another sign that something is amiss with the situation brought about by the new technique. This is not to say that any use of the technique is morally wrong in principle or that it is placing us morally in the wrong as in the case of war, which brings about a situation that is conducive to moral irresponsibility.[11] It is rather to say, as I suggested earlier, that IVF and ET is morally more analogous to divorce which is justifiable in certain circumstances but also confirms a situation that is less than morally desirable because it is not the most conducive to moral responsibility. Thus I have argued that the benefits of the new technique justify its introduction for an initial period of trial at least, but that the problems it brings in its wake, and may bring in the future, from the disappointment of married couples who do not achieve parenthood to the possible dispute about such matters as surrogate motherhood, all betray an environment that is morally problematic. Why should this be so?

The Process of Conception

In my judgement the most important of the issues raised by opponents of IVF and ET is best expressed by reference to the convenantal framework of life.[12] This biblical conception of human existence, and the associated norm of fidelity, indicates that some aspects of human relations are so crucial as to require binding engagements, with a minimum of qualification, on the part of both children and adults. As one would expect, such bonds are expected to govern relations between the sexes and between parents and children and so the introduction of a new means of conceiving children brings with it the question whether or not it seriously disturbs these bonds.

In raising this question about IVF and ET I do not intend to suggest that this technique may be morally wrong because it is contrary to nature. I am inclined to think that systems of morality are human institutions and that those which claim direct dependence upon human nature are mistaken in this respect at least. Nevertheless, the possibility remains that the various institutions or systems of ethics reflect something in 'the nature of things' and derive whatever strength they have precisely from their capacity to order human life in accordance with factors of fundamental importance to human welfare. In his recent set of Gifford Lectures Basil Mitchell refers to the curious modern combination of reluctance to allow such insight to systems of religion and morality and willingness to do so as far as literature is concerned.[13] To say that a system of religion or morality puts people in touch with the nature of things is only to make a modest claim. It need not imply commitment to the belief that the system is absolutely true.

Since a covenant is a binding agreement between at least two parties, even the most rarefied theological version of covenantal ethics must allow for some human influence upon the institution of morality. On the other hand, a more humanistic version will recognize that this influence cannot be arbitrary because the bonds established in certain areas of life relate to matters whose ordering is vital for human welfare. Although the form of these bonds may change over a period of time, then, they require more than a casual fidelity on the part of successive generations. For this reason I would regard the use of IVF and ET for purposes other than the relief of infertility in married couples as morally premature and so unjustified. As for the process itself, my concern is not that conception is caused by other than the 'natural' means of sexual intercourse, but that the intervention of a third party has become, even by comparison with artificial insemination, so direct and all-encompassing that the human bonding which different ethical systems seek to preserve in sex and marriage may be jeopardized. This is what is finally at stake in the actual or potential problems associated with the screening of applicants or the self-knoweldge of progeny.

9 The Created Individual: Are basic notions of humanity threatened?

John L. Morgan

To call an infant born as the result of IVF and ET a 'created' individual is to imply that there is some difference between a child conceived and brought to term in this way and one conceived in the womb (*in vivo*) and carried through completely to term by the mother. Is this kind of distinction justified? To many religious people, and specifically those in the Jewish, Christian, and Islamic traditions, the work of creation belongs, in the first place, to God, as it is outlined in the creation stories of the book of Genesis. God is the one who creates life and order out of chaos. Mankind is the highest product of creation, made from materials which are part of creation. To man, who is made in the image of God, there is given dominion over the created world and the authority to exercise a stewardship which involves caring for what has been created. This has been developed within the Christian tradition so that man may be considered to be a partner with God in the continuing work of creation.

In examining the question of IVF we are not looking at a question of creation out of nothing (*ex nihilo*), but rather what may be seen, from the religious viewpoint, as an aspect of the trust given to mankind to care for creation. It may then be more appropriate to think of the 'facilitated' rather than the 'created' individual when we consider human intervention in the process of human fertilization.

In considering this question and its ramifications we will look at the viewpoints of some writers, both within and outside the Judeo-Christian ethical tradition, and try to determine whether or not basic notions of humanity are threatened by the artificiality which some have claimed is involved in the process.

Those who reject human interference at the beginning of life would almost certainly do so on the basis that what nature has decreed cannot take place ought not to take place. For an infertile couple this implies that they must remain infertile: if they cannot produce a child by the normal means of conception then they must remain childless, they cannot have one 'created' outside the uterus. In this view to take the reproductive materials of the parents, eggs and sperm, and to allow fertilization to take place outside the human body is somehow to dehumanize the resultant product. It is one step short of the Central London Hatchery of Huxley's Brave New World.

To adopt this viewpoint is to take an essentially anti-technology stance: only 'naturally' conceived children are somehow valid. But what is the difference between the two? The answer is usually given in terms of the nature of the conjugal union and its relation to the act of conception. But that is, in part, to say that physical context and not intention is the determinant of status and thus to be conceived as the result of a chance encounter would be regarded as morally superior to a conception that has taken place in a laboratory.

It would seem, however, that the basis of the objections to the use of IVF is not so much because of the present use of the technique as the possibility of practices which will employ it and go further towards the 'creation' of new types of people in a way that is radically different from what is possible at present. The argument here is a consequential one: it is what might happen in the future which is of concern, although frequently this argument is tied in with objections to the technology *per se*.

To allow technological interference at the point of conception is seen as opening the way for designing one's offspring and to open up the possibility of designing the shape (literally) of the next generation and its characteristics. The American Protestant theologian, Paul Ramsey, claims that all reproductive interventions are dehumanizing. He has discussed at length, and in rather polemic fashion, what he thinks will happen to medical ethics and ethics in general when 'the future of the human race is taken to be a patient who is to be reworked by biological technology and through new forms of human reproduction'.[1] He believes that it will, in part, arise from a eugenics policy such as that of Herman J. Muller who, in the 1930s, proposed sperm banks derived from preferred donors to assure the continuance of desirable traits in the human race. Now that the necessary technology is available there does not seem to be any technical reason why one cannot use the sperm of a preferred male donor to fertilize the eggs of a preferred female donor and have the resultant embryo transferred to the host womb of a third person, or even attempt to make use of an artificial placenta. The foetal material could also be stored by freezing and made available later on.

A similar possibility is of course raised by cloning which would seem to represent the most extreme form of technological intervention in the process of reproduction. This is still only a possibility at the human level since the claimed cloning of a human being as reported by the media in 1978 still remains at the level of fiction. Cloning involves the complete absence of insemination and fertilization since the genetic material is taken only from one partner and the result is a genetic mirror image. The aim of this would be to continue features deemed desirable, either by the one whose genetic constitution is to be continued or by society in general, perhaps in an attempt to improve the gene pool as part of a eugenics policy.

Such people who are conceived and born as the results of these practices will, in a sense, be 'created'. One may wonder, however, just how different this kind of creation is from the negative creation practised by parents using the various kinds of technology at present available, ranging from contraception to abortion following amniocentesis so that a malformed child, or one of an undesired sex, may be aborted. If the underlying aim is to create, in the sense of designing one's offspring, then we are already, in some cases, close to doing just that. But between the kinds of practices just mentioned and the use of IVF and re-implantation there is surely a substantial difference. In the present clinical application of these processes all that is being sought is the positive promotion of birth. What could not take place without human technological intervention may now take place. Only to that degree is the resultant offspring 'created'. The objection to the use of IVF at this level seems to be more related to intuitive feelings than to any demonstrable case. If we are prepared to accept the use of some technology within the procreative sphere to enhance, or to impede, the reproductive act, and the amount already employed is fairly great, where should we, if we should, draw the line?

To some Christian ethical thinkers the answer is obvious, as we have already noted in the case of Paul Ramsey. He and other critics of reproductive interventions argue that we should not be masters of our destiny by interfering in this area because human life is a gift which is bestowed by God, and man should not seek to create it artificially. Ramsey insists that the reproductive and love union aspects of sexuality should not, indeed cannot properly, be separated. He rejects the view that such an approach is based 'on a mere biological fact of life, on the "natural law" in this sense, or on Genesis or . . . on the first article of the Creed which speaks of "creation" and the Creator'. Rather, Ramsey finds the basis for his viewpoint in the New Testament, in the Prologue to St John's Gospel, which talks of God creating the world out of love, and from the section on marriage in Chapter 5 of St Paul's Epistle to the Ephesians, which discusses the love which should exist between husbands and wives. According to him, 'these two passages point to one and the same Lord — the Lord who presides over procreation as well as the lord of all marital covenants — the two aspects of human sexuality belong together . . . not simply because they are found together in human and other animal bisexual reproduction'. Because Ramsey gives to the relationship of male and female an end — a *telos* — outside the fact of the relationship itself, or outside simple procreation, that end being Christ, he is able to conclude:

> To put radically asunder what God joined together in parenthood when He made love procreative, to procreate beyond the sphere of love (AID, for example, or making human life in a test-tube), or to posit acts of sexual love beyond the sphere of responsible creation (by definition, marriage), means a refusal of the image of God's creation in our own.[2]

On the other hand, the humanist, and some Christians will argue that 'man is a maker and a selector and a designer and the more rationally contrived and deliberate anything is, the more human it is'. On this basis it would be possible to claim of laboratory reproduction, or laboratory assisted reproduction, that it is 'radically human compared to conception by ordinary human intercourse. It is willed, chosen, purposed, and controlled, and surely these are amongst the traits that distinguish *homo sapiens* from others in the animal genus'.[3]

This is the doyen of Christian situationist ethicists, Joseph Fletcher, arguing from a particular understanding of the normatively human. It begins with an *a priori* assumption of what that is, and it is the initial assumption which determines the outcome. Those who argue against this viewpoint also begin with an assumption but one regarding the inherent naturalness of the normal form of conception. A non-religious critic of IVF, a biologist, Dr Leon Kass, claims that 'there are more or less human ways of bringing a child into the world. I am arguing that the laboratory procreation of human beings is no longer *human* procreation'.[4]

In his approach an assumption and an intuitive feeling about the inherent superiority of 'natural' conception are fused together. The act of conception is thus regarded as a mystery into which the scientist should not intrude too deeply. It would seem that Dr Kass would draw the line for human and technological intervention at pre-fertilization. A child conceived *in vitro* would be the result not only of rational technical planning, but also of a non-emotional experience. Accompanying the conception and birth of such a child there will be too little of the 'mystery of nature'. Parenting, to borrow a theological term, will have become demythologized. Kass's approach is not far short of some aspects of Ramsey's viewpoint, although without the specifically religious element.

The basis of traditional Roman Catholic objections to reproductive interventions involves the severing of the link between love and the sexual act at conception. When Pope Pius XII condemned artificial insemination in an address at the Second World Congress on Fertility and Sterility, he took an essentially natural law approach:

A child is the fruit of conjugal union when this union is fully expressed by the bringing into play of the organic functions and the sensory emotions attached to them, and of the spiritual and disinterested love which animates this union. It is in the unity of this human act that the biological conditions of generation must be posited.

This was obviously the rationale for his prohibition of IVF, which he condemned *a fortiori* in the same address saying 'On the subject of attempts at artificial human fecundation "*in vitro*"', let it suffice for us to state that such attempts must be rejected as immoral and absolutely unlawful'.[5]

The objections by Pope Pius XII and Dr Kass are to laboratory-aided fertilization, to the intrustion of external agents into the process of the generation of life and underlying this there is also a fear. Dr Kass expresses it strongly: 'To lay one's hands on human generations is to take a major step toward man making himself another of the man-made things'.[6] The man made is in this view not only inferior but also threatening since it is ultimately seen as dehumanizing.

What also underlies, in an ethical sense, the objection to the technical cultural interference in human reproduction which is said to dehumanize? Is there possibly something further implied by the 'wisdom in that mystery of nature which joins the pleasure of sex, the communication of love and the desire for children' as expressed by Kass, or a child as 'the fruit of disinterested and spiritual love' as described by Pope Pius?

There are two possible points which have been made regarding this underlying ethical basis, apart from any biological objections, which may also have ethical import. Daniel Callahan has suggested that these objections may be related to 'the establishment of those bonds and values which serve to facilitate two human goods'.[7] First, the biological act of begetting is directed towards the creation of a sense of obligation, which is the very basis of community. This begins in, and is exemplified by, the parent-child relationship. Secondly, there is the specific responsibility of particular adults for their own children which stems in part from the natural and concrete parent-child relationship. The biological and affectional basis reinforces or facilitates an irrevocable commitment. Callahan thinks that this is what Kass might have had in mind. If a child is 'created' by technological intervention what is the responsibility of the scientist? Is he, as Kass seems to suggest, a new kind of parent, and what does that mean in terms of relationships? Will reproductive intervention weaken the traditional bonds of parent and child in such a way that we will eventually see a new pattern of socialization emerging and eventually a new kind of society?

We have not yet had many studies of the lives of AID-conceived children, who are, in some ways analogous. What little information that is available does not, so far, seem to suggest any serious difficulties. In the case of IVF-conceived children, where the biological parents are also the social parents, this would seem to make the development of difficulties or new types of relationships even less likely. It is after all out of mutual love and a desire for creativity within marriage that IVF procedures are initiated by the parents using their own reproductive materials.

In IVF the objection is to the facilitation of conception by an external agent using a developed technology. The crux of the objection is that it takes place outside the body and the sexual act. If IVF is to be regarded as 'inhuman' or 'dehumanizing', the objection must be based here.

As we have seen, however, one school of thought would argue strongly that it is precisely because of this, that by the use of a technique such as IVF assisting in the work of creation we actually assert our humanity: therefore the child so conceived must perforce be human. If it is, in part, theologically inspired criticisms which have supported the view that it is dehumanizing, then we must probe a little more deeply the normative view of the human which goes to the opposite pole and is able to see the use of technology, even in the most personal of areas, as characteristically human.

Throughout history mankind has developed technologies of various kinds, and it is this capacity for innovative development which has entered into our very definition of the difference between animals and human beings. Often this inventiveness has brought with it great benefits for the race as a whole, but it must also be acknowledged that sometimes it has been used for wrong ends. The beneficial inventiveness of man, however, is for some a part of the definition of the normatively human; it is a use of the stewardship that is given to humans and it is not a closed option. This view contrasts with a more static view of the human, which sees the meaning of humanity as rather more a given one and which would stress the place of pride (*hubris*) in the human make-up. This invites suspicion concerning all human ventures and would tend to be restrictive in an *a priori* way about what one could do in the biomedical field, both in terms of the means that may be employed as well as the ends that may be sought.[7] In this view morality is imposed, since the human is defined from without in an authoritative fashion.

The view which sees inventiveness and innovation as characteristically human does not rush to the opposite extreme and 'baptize' every new development or proposal in, for example, the medical area. It recognizes that we may legitimately interfere with nature, including our own. The power of self-creation is seen as a legitimate gift from God. This was recognized by Thomas Aquinas when he saw 'man as an image of God' precisely because he is 'endowed with intelligence, free will, and a power of his actions which is proper to him . . . having dominion over his own activities'.[8] It is the development of this kind of view which gives a limited licence to interfere with the normal process of reproduction to the extent of using IVF to help in the characteristic human way of procreation. This technology utilizes man's creativeness and his capacity for self-creation of which Karl Rahner wrote: 'human self-creation means quite simply that today man is changing himself. To be more precise: man is consciously and deliberately changing himself."[9]

In the biomedical field this 'changing' may be equated with the power to intervene to accomplish that which was previously impossible, in this case, by the accomplishment of conception and bringing to term of an infant remarkable only for the extrauterine manner of the conception. The processes involved here will not affect the status of the child or dehumanize the reproductive process.

The foregoing is not the same as the blanket endorsement given by some thinkers to whatever it is that scientists would wish to do in this field. This tends to be the approach of what might be called the 'over-optimistic' school. Joseph Fletcher goes too far in this direction when dealing with the question of the artificiality or otherwise of laboratory-assisted reproduction:

Men are characterized by technique, and for a human being to oppose technology is self-hatred. We are often confused on this score, attitudinally. A 'test-tube baby', for example, although conceived and gestated '*ex corpo*', would nonetheless be humanly reproduced and of human value. A baby made artificially, by deliberate and careful contrivance, would be more human than one resulting from sexual roulette — the reproductive mode of the human species.[10]

Such an approach gives too much weight to cultural factors and pays too little attention to more basic values involved in the realms of science and medicine where they impinge upon cherished institutions. It is one thing to allow the use of IVF where a married couple cannot conceive by themselves; this may be seen as an appropriate use of technology and not be regarded as dehumanizing, but Fletcher's understanding of the normatively human begins at the wrong end. There is a constant danger that technology will carry its imperatives and that sooner or later what can be done will be done regardless. When this point is reached our humanity would be endangered.

The constant concern of those who are cautious about endorsing the use of IVF is that a technique which is used to overcome a physical defect will provide such a breach of the normal method of procreation that because it is efficient and can be controlled it will come to replace that which is valued for a totally different set of reasons, which are believed to be closer to the heart of what is distinctively human.

Given the present costs and the availability of medical resources involved in such practices, this kind of anxiety would not seem well founded. Parents untroubled by infertility will continue to conceive their children and mothers to gestate them in the normal way. We must recognize, however, that there will be always those for whom the technologically novel has a certain appeal, or who may be attracted by the idea of a method which would guarantee a successful pregnancy. It would seem desirable that there should be fairly explicit guidelines developed for experimentation in this area, and for the now more or less regularized techniques which are involved in IVF. Any threats of a wide-scale assault on characteristically human values and institutions will come from developments of techniques which make use of IVF in cloning, genetic engineering, or using artificial placentae for gestation outside the body. These may be seen as creating human life but in a way that is very different from the present application of IVF, which has re-implantation, rather than ET, as its goal.

The separation of the union of the sexual act and conception in procreation is not a neutral thing. As Richard McCormick puts it: 'The artificial route to pregnancy is a disvalue and one that needs justification.'[11] It would seem, however, that the integrity of the procreative process is not attacked by IVF, where the embryo conceived is the expression and embodiment of love, since the child is the result of a decision from within the procreative context of husband and wife. At this point technology is simply being used in the service of humanity and need not threaten or diminish it, unless we exchange an ethic of responsibility for one of irresponsibility in our exercise of creativity.

10 Surrogate Motherhood: The position and problems of substitutes

*Alan A. Rassaby**

And still Abram's wife Sarai bore him no children. But she had an Egyptian maid-servant, called Agar; and now she said to her husband, The Lord, as thou seest, denies me motherhood; Betake thyself to this maid of mine, in the hope that I may at least have children through her means.

Genesis 16

For most of us, the term 'surrogate motherhood' is so closely associated with the 'new technology' that the idea that it has been going on for many thousands of years could come as something of a shock. It could also prove professionally embarrassing to an army of journalists[1] who have so recently and loudly trumpeted the advent of a fresh challenge to our old values. One can sympathize with the journalist who regards the tale of Abram, Sarai, and Agar with a measure of suspicion, after all, it is not exactly current news. At the same time, it takes us closer to the heart of the matter.

For the word 'surrogate' means no more than 'substitute'. A surrogate mother is a substitute mother: she is a person who, for financial or compassionate reasons, agrees to bear a child for someone else. A couple could conceivably enlist the services of a surrogate mother because the female partner is unable or unwilling either to become

*Alan Rassaby wishes to acknowledge the support of the Myer Foundation of Australia.

pregnant or to carry a pregnancy to term. A woman who suffers from a heart disease or partial paralysis or who has a history of miscarriages could fall within this category.

For many of these couples, adoption is no longer a viable alternative because of the age of one or both of the applicants or because of the diminishing numbers of healthy, non-handicapped babies who are available for adoption.

Surrogate motherhood has until now taken one of two forms. In its first form, the husband of a woman may impregnate a second woman by means of sexual intercourse (as in the story of Abram). On birth of the child, the surrogate relinquishes custody of the child to the couple and according to the terms of an earlier agreement or contract under which she may receive certain financial benefits.

In its second and more publicized form, the impregnation occurs through a process of artificial insemination. This method avoids the 'adultery aspect' present in the first variant while still satisfying the desires of a certain number of couples to have a child who is at least partially biologically their own.

Lawyers exploring the legality of these arrangements find that they must navigate hitherto uncharted water. Rapid technological advances in the IVF programme may soon force them further adrift. It may soon be possible for a couple to 'have' a child which is totally biologically their own without the child's 'mother' ever giving birth. In this third form of surrogate motherhood, the ovum of a woman could be fertilized with the sperm of her husband through a process of IVF and transplanted in the body of another woman, who would then bear no genetic relationship to the child to which she would give birth. For the lawyer who attempts to resolve a dispute between on the one hand the child's genetic mother and on the other the child's birth-giving mother (the surrogate), the new technology adds an unwelcome dimension to an already complex issue.

In this chapter, I propose to explore the legal and ethical issues which arise out of surrogate motherhood with special reference to the third form and to the new dimension which it adds to the problem.

The Present State of the Law

Let us assume that X gives birth to a baby who is genetically the child of Y and Z. X can be described as the child's surrogate mother and Y and Z as the child's genetic parents. The surrogate mother no longer wishes to honour an agreement which was signed by the three parties before her pregnancy. She refuses to relinquish custody of the child to the genetic parents. What legal recourse would the genetic parents then have? A lawyer acting for them could seek to establish that the genetic, and not the surrogate, mother is the legal mother of the baby and that therefore she is the person who is entitled to immediate custody. This proposition is a simple one based on the well-established legal right which a mother has to custody of her child. It has nothing whatsoever to do with the question of whether the contract entered into by the parties is legally enforceable.

Who is the Child's Mother?

A judge who is required to resolve a dispute over the identity of the child's legal mother would have three options open to him. Either the surrogate is the child's mother and the genetic mother is not or the genetic mother is the mother and the surrogate is not or both of them are joint mothers. The choice which the judge makes is likely to have a significant effect on the operation of the law. The person who can establish that she is the child's legal mother to the exclusion of all others will have established a legal right to custody unless the exercise by her of that right would not be in the best interests of the child.[1] If the judge favours the genetic mother, the child can be said to be the nuptial child of the genetic parents, but if the judge accepts the proposition asserted by the surrogate mother, the child would be the ex-nuptial child of the surrogate mother and the genetic father and would consequently share with other ex-nuptial children certain legal disabilities.

On which criteria should a judge base his decision? The most likely yardstick would be biological input. To what extent could the child be said to be the biological product of one woman rather than the other? The genetic mother would no doubt point out that the child's genetic blueprint is immutably fixed at the time of fertilization. She may argue that any effect which the surrogate mother has on the developing foetus must therefore be considered a minimal one. In this respect, her argument would be enhanced by the fact that the foetus, because it is a foreign body with a different blood system from that of the surrogate, would not be affected directly by the presence or absence of particular antibodies in the blood system of the surrogate mother. The genetic mother may also contend, with some justification, that a child with the genes for dark hair and short, stocky stature will not be any fairer, taller or slimmer for having been born of a woman with these genetic characteristics.

On the other hand, the surrogate mother is certainly more than an insulator or oven. The growing foetus will depend on her for nutrition and the removal of waste products. If the surrogate mother is malnourished or an alcoholic, the foetus is likely to suffer adversely. Smoking has been identified with smaller infants at birth[2] and the effects of various drugs on the central nervous system, such as Thalidomide, have been well documented.[3] In addition there are numerous other socio-economic, demographic, and maternal medical factors which can contribute to a high risk pregnancy with an increased chance of death or disability to the foetus.[4]

All of which suggests that although both the genetic and surrogate mothers would be able to point to cogent evidence indicating that each is the child's biological mother, *ipso facto* neither would succeed in establishing that the other was not the biological mother. In the words of one legal writer, 'the revered institution of motherhood appears to be divisible, and has the potential . . . to be undertaken as a collaborative enterprise'.[5] Biologically, it seems that the child would indeed have two mothers, a possibility already adverted to by at least one theologian.[6] In view of this, 'it would be inappropriate for a lawyer to attempt to balance these two arguments and come to any fixed conclusion'.[7]

Assuming that there is a parent-child relationship with both 'mothers', then the question of which mother should have legal custody remains to be resolved on other considerations. Other questions of law also remain unanswered. Which mother is to be responsible for the child's education and medical care? Which mother is required to register the birth of the child?[8] Which mother is obliged by law to make adequate provision in her will for the child's proper maintenance and support?[9]

Is the Contract Enforceable?

Finding that the question of maternal identity tends to obscure rather than clarify the legal issues, the genetic mother may then seek to establish that she has a legally enforceable right to custody of the child on the basis of a valid and binding contract. This is the second string to her bow. All the hallmarks of a legally binding contract may be present, including the making of an offer to the surrogate mother, the acceptance of that offer by her, and valuable consideration (being a promise to pay the surrogate mother a certain sum of money in return for a promise on her part to relinquish custody of the child). Even so, the contract will not be enforceable if it is against public policy, that is, if it is injurious to society.

Is a 'surrogacy contract' injurious to society? Although there can be no direct legal precedent, a study of analogous case law in England and the United States can give us some insight into the relevant legal principles. The body of cases may conveniently be divided into older cases and newer cases. The older cases involved questions of the legality of contractual arrangements whereby parents of a child had agreed to relinquish custody in favour of some other person in return for some financial gain to themselves or to the child in question. The newer cases dealt with the legal enforceability of contractual arrangements entered into between a surrogate mother and the child's father (and sometimes his wife), where the latter's sperm had been used to impregnate the surrogate through a process of artificial insemination. I have earlier referred to this as the second form of surrogate motherhood.

The scant English authority in the area would seem to justify the proposition that, in that country, a contract by a parent to transfer parental rights and liabilities to another person will always be unenforceable on the grounds that it is against public policy.[10] In the United States, the principle has not always been stated so widely.[11] The following statements, however, appear to be true statements of the law in the United States, and they apply equally in English law:

- A transaction which amounts to the sale of a child is contrary to public policy.[12]
- A court has never enforced any contract where enforcement means that legal custody of a child would pass from one person to another.

The first of the 'new wave' cases occurred in England in 1978. A and B, an unmarried couple, wished to employ the services of C to have a child. C was artificially inseminated with B's sperm. The agreement was that C would relinquish custody of the child on birth in return for which she would receive £500. C later refused to honour the agreement. A and B sought custody of the child through the courts. The presiding judge refused to enforce the agreement on the basis that it was no more than a contract for the sale and purchase of a child and that as such it was 'pernicious' and unenforceable.[13]

In an apparent departure from these principles, a Kentucky judge recently sanctioned a similar contract. In that case, a childless couple from Illinois entered into a contract with a woman who was willing to act as a surrogate mother. As in the English case, the surrogate was artificially inseminated with the sperm of the male member of the couple and agreed to relinquish custody of the child on receipt of a fee. In contrast to that case, however, the surrogate did fulfil her part of the bargain. The presiding judge ruled that this constituted a valid mode of adoption and that the child's father and his wife were entitled to claim legal parenthood.[14] It is thought that Kentucky's attorney-general may challenge this decision.[15]

Given the principles established by the older body of case law, it seems unlikely that the Kentucky decision was correctly decided.[16] Certainly an Australian court would be more likely to follow the English example in preference to the Kentucky one. It is therefore probably correct to say that a genetic mother of a child would not win legal custody by attempting to establish that she had a contractual agreement with the child's birth-giving mother.

The Need for a New Approach

Even if one could resolve the equivocal legal status of the child by reference to well-established legal principles, the fact remains that one would thereby impose on the community a rule or set of rules designed for another period of history. The law must surely be re-assessed to take into account changing needs and changing phenomena. Any legislation which is enacted will thereby reflect a thorough consideration of the ethical and social perspectives of the problem. Law makers must ask whether surrogacy is acceptable and, if so, whether its use should be regulated in some way.

Is Surrogacy Acceptable?

An analysis of the surrogacy debate reveals the existence of four schools of thought. In the first school are those who believe that surrogacy should be proscribed because it constitutes an unacceptable practice. In the second are those who argue that a person who has given birth to a child should not be legally forced to relinquish custody of that child to another person with whom she has contracted. A proponent of this view may or may not believe that surrogacy should be encouraged because of its positive aspects. Finally, there are those people who believe that surrogacy is inevitable and that society must protect itself and its members by regulating the process. Supporters of this alternative see no point in debating the merits or otherwise of surrogacy. Their attitude is best expressed in the words 'it's here to stay, so let's do our best with what we've got'.

Subscribers to the first view raise a number of objections to surrogacy. Some would argue that it encourages immorality. Dickens observes that 'a female who, especially but not only for payment, offers the services of her body for the gratification of others is so quickly vilified and named as a whore that consideration of reputable and modern analogues for the practice of embryo transfer must consciously be sought'.

To adopt this view would be to ignore the wealth of existing analogues. The wet nurse who provides milk for the suckling infant and the person who donates a kidney or other organ for use in a transplant operation are but two such samples. Nor are biblical analogues inappropriate. Just as Sarai sought to satisfy her desire for maternity through her maid-servant, Agar, so too did the barren Rachel give her maid-servant, Bala, to the Patriach Jacob in order that 'through her means, I shall have a family of my own' (Genesis 30). Certainly in the biblical context, a woman who volunteered to have a child for another woman, far from being vilified, was blessed.

Others argue that to sanction surrogacy would be to encourage exploitation of both the surrogate and the person who seeks her services. The latter could be charged vast and unconscionable sums for these services. This would hardly seem to be a good reason to proscribe surrogacy but instead reminds us of the need for government regulation of the transaction. More commonly, ethicists object to surrogacy on the ground that the surrogate herself could be coerced into that role through poverty or unemployment.[18] From one perspective, the surrogate can conceivably be regarded as the victim of an unfair social order. Without denying this, it seems rather counterproductive to deny her this option. Given a choice between poverty and exploitation, many people may prefer the latter. The dilemma recalls to mind the words of a friend who told me that she never gives money to intellectually handicapped children collecting from the occupants of stationary cars at traffic lights because they were underpaid and exploited by the charities that employed them. I wonder to where else these children could have looked for a source of income.

Another proposition sometimes asserted is that surrogacy may prove to be against the interests of both the surrogate mother who gives up the child and the child himself or herself. Little research has been done on the psychological and emotional bonds that tie a child to its 'birth-giving' mother and the trauma which could result on separation. If we continue to permit adoption, however, we can hardly ban surrogacy on this ground.

The primary benefit of surrogacy is that it would satisfy the desires and perceived needs of a number of women including those women who are unable to carry a child to term and who cannot adopt a baby because of advancing age or for some other reason. For those people, access to the services of a surrogate will become increasingly important as the numbers of babies available for adoption continue to decline.[19] It is this social service factor which persuades me that surrogacy should be a legitimate practice. I do not think that the surrogate's receiving payment for the service detracts from its social value in any way. Nor am I persuaded by the argument that the children will be 'devalued' in the eyes of the community because they are 'bought and sold'. In most cases, the services of a surrogate will only be sought after all other viable alternatives have been exhausted. Far from being devalued, this child is likely to be especially loved.

Leaving aside the positive and negative aspects of surrogacy, there are good grounds for the belief that people who are desperate enough in their desire to have a child, and who cannot do so by natural methods, will not obey a proscription anyway. If this is true, to proscribe surrogacy would be only to force the practice 'underground' and to deny ourselves the opportunity to regulate the procedure to the benefit of both parties, the child, and society. In this sense, an interdiction of surrogacy may be likened to a prohibition of alcohol. Of course, it may be possible to proscribe ET to surrogates, thereby prohibiting one form of surrogacy. The technical aspects of this procedure are so complex and its availability so limited in consequence that the prohibition would be likely to be complete. This is one form only of surrogacy, however, and will always remain a small part of it. The question of whether surrogacy should be permissible must be seen in the broader context. From this perspective, the law may never succeed in prohibiting surrogacy agreements. Instead, law makers must look to appropriate methods of regulating the practice.

On Regulating Surrogacy

A central theme in the debate over regulation is whether access to the services of a surrogate should be restricted to those people who, for medical reasons, are unable to bear a child and should be denied to those women who, though physically capable of giving birth, do not do so either because they are too busy or because their careers require certain aesthetic standards which would not be met if they were pregnant. Lawyers have expressed conflicting views on this matter.[20]

I do not believe that we are entitled to argue (as some have argued) that the need of the woman who physically cannot give birth is an actual one whereas the need of the busy female executive or model is more perceived than actual. To the latter, the need may be just as great as to the former. Unfortunately, one can expect there to be some discrimination in practice, however, at least in times of scarce resources. One cannot avoid the fact that society places a greater premium on a woman's childbearing role than it does on her employment prospects. A woman who physically cannot give birth will therefore be regarded with more sympathy and will be perceived to have a greater need than the woman whose vocational ambitions preclude a natural childbirth.

Another question to which consideration should be given is that of payment for the services of the surrogate. Should the parties be able to negotiate a price on a free enterprise basis or should the law regulate this aspect of the transaction by setting a recommended and a maximum fee for services? The potential for exploitation of both parties persuades me that the latter is the preferable option.

Of great importance is the need for the responsibilities of both parties to be clearly set out at the time at which the agreement is signed. Law makers must consider whether or not the surrogate mother should be responsible for any medical costs incurred during her pregnancy or whether this should be the responsibility of the genetic mother of the child. Complications during pregnancy may result in serious illness requiring a lengthy period of hospitalization. In such cases, the costs of health care or subsequent loss of income or both may be substantial. Consideration should be given, therefore, to the inclusion of a compulsory insurance scheme in the terms of every agreement. The genetic mother (or the surrogate) may be obliged to pay the premiums on the scheme.

The identity of the surrogate is also a matter of importance. Should the surrogate be required to pass a medical fitness test before and during pregnancy? Should she be required to undergo psychological assessment? Should the surrogate be forced to retire at a certain age?

One matter which clearly demands regulation is the activities of the surrogate mother during pregnancy. Should she be prohibited from smoking or drinking alcohol? What about activities which are potentially (though not intrinsically) harmful, for example, skiing? At what point does regulation become unfairly intrusive on the lives of the surrogates? What if the baby is born with a disability which can be directly attributed to an activity in which the surrogate mother engaged which was in breach of the agreement (or in breach of the law)? In such a case, should the child or his or her genetic parents have a right of action in negligence (or breach of statutory duty) against the surrogate mother?

Some writers have also discussed whether the surrogate could and should be compelled to submit to amniocentesis, and whether she can be constrained to undergo an abortion if the procedure indicates some birth defect or if the genetic parents have simply changed their minds and no longer wish to have a child.[21] At present, legal compulsion without the consent of the surrogate would not be possible.[22]

At the epicentre of the dilemma is whether a surrogate mother should be legally compellable to relinquish custody of a child in favour of his or her genetic parent(s). It is one thing to recognize that a person may validly relinquish control of a child to another person who then assumes parental responsibilities in relation to the child. It is another proposition entirely to suggest that the person should be compelled to do so.

Those who believe that the surrogate should not be compellable compare surrogacy with adoption. They point out that in many jurisdictions, a parent is allowed a period of time following the birth of the child during which consent to adoption may be revoked. In Victoria, Australia, the period is thirty days. In this way, the natural mother has a period of time during which to reconsider her decision and either come to terms with it or revoke it. They argue that a similar law in the surrogacy context is desirable if adequate consideration is to be given to the trauma which the surrogate would be likely to suffer if compelled to relinquish custody of the child.

Those who assert that the surrogate should be compellable dispute the value of the adoption analogy. They point out that in the adoption context, the potential adoptive parent can have no legitimate expectation of or moral right to custody of a particular child because he or she has no contractual arrangement (or arrangement of any kind) with the natural parent, nor does he or she contribute in any way to the birth. In contrast, the genetic parent in the surrogacy context does enter into a contractual arrangement and does make a significant contribution by providing the surrogate with an ovum without which the child could never have been born. They argue further that if the surrogate is not compellable, surrogacy contracts will be breached with impunity.

The solution may be a compromise. Arguably, the long-term emotional trauma suffered by a surrogate mother who unwillingly relinquishes custody of her child may be so great that the law should adopt a special attitude to this type of contract by refusing to compel the surrogate to relinquish custody. If this is so, the law may still recognize the legitimate claim of the child's genetic mother by imposing a penalty on a surrogate who fails to fulfil her part of the bargain. Alternatively, a surrogate may be asked to leave a valuable deposit with a person or body agreed upon by both parties. The deposit could be forfeited in the event of a breach by the surrogate mother.

A much neglected facet of the debate is the issue of a right to privacy. At present, people who seek the services of a surrogate must usually enter into direct negotiations with the surrogate. Because the identity of all parties is known, privacy may become a source of great difficulty. A surrogate who changes her mind at some later stage and who comes to 'claim' her child could cause incalculable emotional distress and damage to the child and to his or her present 'parents'. For this reason, I believe that all surrogacy contracts should be arranged through a surrogacy agency. The intervention of an agency would mean that the surrogate and the person seeking her services would have no direct contact with one another. Each would therefore remain ignorant of the identity of the other. It is essential, of course, that the agency keep a proper register of the transaction, which includes the names of all parties involved.

The agency would also serve a number of other useful functions. Agency staff could provide a counselling service to the three parties. People who seek the services of a surrogate could be advised of practical alternatives, and the person willing to act as surrogate could be prepared for the task and also psychologically (and medically) assessed to determine her suitability. This task could be undertaken with the help of women who have already acted as surrogate mothers. Older children and adults who are experiencing difficulty in coming to terms with the circumstances of their birth could receive valuable help from agency counsellors.

At the same time, the lessons learned in the adoption context should not be forgotten. Agency involvement should guarantee privacy but not unqualified secrecy. A person has a moral right to have access to any personal information about himself or herself. Genetic parents should inform the child at a very early age of the circumstances of birth to avoid any trauma associated with unintended discovery.[23] When the child reached the age of majority, he or she should have a legal right to acquire a copy of a birth certificate or agency record containing the name of the surrogate mother. Literature in this area is strongly supportive of the view that access to such information is likely to be beneficial to the child because it may satisfy an often long-felt desire to establish or complete a sense of true self-identity and may also facilitate a closer relationship with the genetic parents without causing an appreciable invasion of the privacy of or trauma to the surrogate mother.[24]

The Next Step

Law makers must now choose between three options. First of all, they can ignore the storm which is gathering around the surrogacy debate and leave questions of legality to be determined on existing common law and statutory principles. Secondly, they can proscribe surrogacy by means of legislation. Thirdly, they can legislate to permit surrogacy either absolutely or subject to certain restrictions.

The first alternative is both short-sighted and impractical. It is impractical because the existing law is far from clear in its implications. It is short-sighted because it fails to take into account that a society with new technology and changing values deserves a fresh approach to questions of law reform and not one which is basted in the values of another time.

The second alternative ignores some of the benefits which surrogacy may bring. It is probably also unrealistic because it represents an attempt to proscribe what is arguably an inevitable event. Such a proscription could moreover force the practice 'underground' thereby increasing the potential for exploitation.

I believe that the solution lies in careful and detailed legislative regulation designed to promote the interests of all parties and of our society in general. One hopes that the process of law reform is set in train well before the problems grow to unmanageable proportions.

11 Cloning, Ectogenesis, and Hybrids: Things to come?

William A. W. Walters

IVF and ET for the treatment of infertility almost pale into insignificance in the minds of many when suggestions, however tentative and exploratory, are made about cloning, ectogenesis, and hybridization. Although these procedures have not yet been used in man, the possibility in the not too distant future raises much anxiety or even fear about the future of humanity, which may or may not be warranted.

In a sense, the success of IVF and ET in man paves the way for related techniques such as those which form the subjects of this chapter. It behoves me, therefore, to consider these techniques and their ethical implications seriously before they are used in man for whatever reasons.

Cloning

The word 'clone' comes from the Greek, *klon*, meaning a young shoot or twig, and in cell biology refers to a group of cells, each member of which has developed from a single parent cell. The term was originally used by plant biologists, and the cutting taken from a plant which grows into a new plant having identical characteristics with its parent is a form of cloning. This is an essential feature of cloning, that the individual member cells of a clone are identical with one another and with the parent cell.

Theoretically, the procedure of cloning is simple. The nucleus of a mature unfertilized egg cell is removed by microsurgery or irradiation and replaced by a nucleus obtained from a body cell (other than a germ cell) of an adult organism of the same species. Such nucleus-donor cells could be obtained from the skin, intestinal tract, respiratory tract, and so on. An extraordinary event now takes place. The egg cell develops as if it had been fertilized in the usual manner by a sperm cell, and a new organism is produced with a genetic constitution identical with that of the parent of the donated cell nucleus. Thus reproduction has been achieved by asexual rather than sexual means. The mechanism of this is not yet understood.

Cloning provides a striking contrast to sexual reproduction which results in offspring that are genetically different from each parent as a result of mixing and recombination of genes at fertilization. Thus the new individual resulting from sexual reproduction has a mixture of genes, 50 per cent of maternal and 50 per cent of paternal origin. A gene is the basic unit of inheritance consisting of a specific length of de-oxy-ribonucleic acid (DNA). The latter comprises the hereditary material of the cell and is located in the chromosomes of the nucleus. Genes direct the production of specific proteins that are characteristic for the cell concerned and its function. On the other hand, the asexual reproduction of cloning results in the new individual having all of the genes of one parent only. Indeed, it should be emphasized that all members of a clone have an identical genetic constitution except for mutations that may occur. A mutation is a physiochemical change in the character of a gene, which in effect gives rise to a new or mutant gene.

Although cloning has been used with varying success in frogs, salamanders, and fruit flies, it has not yet been successful in higher animals or man. The report by David Rorvik,[1] a journalist, claiming that a businessman had had himself cloned has not been substantiated, and several distinguished biological scientists have expressed an opinion that the state of the art is not yet far enough advanced to make such a report credible. Cloning is still a technically difficult procedure especially with the microscopic-sized eggs of mammals and man compared with the relatively large eggs of frogs, which can be seen readily with the naked eye. Even when frogs are cloned, Gurdon[2] in Oxford found that only 1 to 2 per cent of the cloned eggs developed into normal tadpoles and then frogs. In addition, an appreciable number of seriously abnormal embryos were produced and the majority of the eggs failed to undergo embryonic develop-ment. With such high risks of abnormal embryos, it is obvious that much more research will be required before the techniques can be safely used in mammals and man.

Another type of cloning is embryo fission. This involves separating the cells of an early embryo at the two-cell stage and transplanting each of them into a recipient uterus, suitably primed hormonally, where they can develop into complete and genetically identical embryos. This technique has been applied to mouse embryos up to the eight-cell stage, but beyond this the cells seem to have lost their ability to develop into new embryos.[3]

Unlike nuclear transfer cloning, embryo fission does not allow one to select the genetic prototype unless one has already used nuclear transfer to obtain the embryo in question.

Cloning raises a number of ethical issues which can be discussed in terms of objections and assent.

The clonee, or individual produced by cloning, may at some stage be told that his genetic constitution is the same as that of an identifiable living person. This knowledge could have a deleterious psychological effect on the child especially if he recognized some physical or mental characteristics of his parent that he did not like. Consequently, he may become depressed or behave in an antisocial manner.

This hypothetical argument could also apply, however, in the case of a child conceived in the normal manner, who might feel just as antagonistic to his parents for bringing him into existence if he took exception to characteristics of either parent for one reason or another.

It is also obvious that if the cloned child happened to like the characteristics of his parent, he would be pleased with the nature of his conception.

Another cause for concern is the suggestion that the creation of multiple copies of one person, namely the nucleus donor, may lead to loss of identity in the clonees. The latter might feel a lack of the sense of uniqueness or self when confronted by others of identical genotype.[4] But as Mackay[5] points out this argument fails to recognize that what distinguishes one human being from another is basically the unique pattern of roles and relationships he bears among his fellows and not any dissimilarity of his body from theirs.

Furthermore, identical twins are known to be particularly close to one another emotionally and psychologically rather than lacking a sense of uniqueness or self. In any case, it is not necessarily desirable to emphasize the self, when one considers this in the light of the teachings of Buddha, Jesus Christ, and other religious leaders, who were at pains to teach the necessity of eradication of feelings of self. In this context, it could be argued that clonees would co-operate better with one another and others precisely because of this lack of a sense of self.

Another ethical concern is with the problem of laboratory mistakes during cloning. If foetal abnormalities result which are compatible with life but likely to render the individual severely handicapped either mentally or physically, what is to be done? As long as the abnormality was detected early enough in pregnancy, termination of pregnancy could be offered. Currently this occurs when foetal abnormalities are detected *in utero* by various antenatal intrauterine diagnostic tests. The essential difference between these two situations, ethically, is that in the former the abnormality has occurred as a result of deliberate human experimentation, whereas in the latter it has resulted from a chance factor in normal reproduction. In reply to this objection to cloning, it may be expected that mistakes of this nature would be much less likely to occur if cloning techniques were first established in various animals including primates before being tried in man.

Ramsey[6] and a number of ethicists have suggested that cloning is such an impersonal process that it threatens to undermine the human and personal elements in parenthood. As only one parent of either sex would be necessary, this could reduce men to a feeling of being castrated or women to a feeling of being mere incubators,[7] depending upon the sex of the person who donated the body cell nucleus. To separate reproduction from the sphere of bodily love and sexual union is likely to have a dehumanizing effect, according to some.[8] Consequently, the breakdown of the family and wider society would inevitably occur. The same theoretical objections apply to IVF and ET for relief of infertility, but our experience in Melbourne with ten successful pregnancies from this type of conception has been to the contrary. Because the couples concerned wanted a child so desperately, and because the husband has been encouraged to accompany his wife during each phase of the IVF procedure, the result has been to increase their love and concern for one another and for the conceptus. The latter has not come into being as a result of gratification of sexual desire as is often the case with normal human reproduction, when pregnancy may be not only unplanned but unwanted. On the contrary, the pregnancy has been planned, wanted, and loved from the very beginning.

Inevitably, cloning incorporates sex determination and raises concern about a disturbance of the balance of the sexes. If, for any reason, one sex becomes predominant, it may mean that adverse societal effects would result.

It has also been postulated that cloning along with all other artificial reproductive procedures will lead to a lack of respect for the sanctity and dignity of human life,[9] presumably particularly among the technologists involved. This postulate may be based upon the old adage 'familiarity breeds contempt'. Common conditions, however, occur commonly in medical practice and yet there is no evidence that medical practitioners are less concerned about their patients with such conditions.

There is a danger that cloned people may not be as adaptable with the passage of time to a changing environment as their fellows originating from sexual reproduction. The latter is an important means of ensuring genetic adaptability. Furthermore, if cloned people chose to return to sexual reproduction after several generations of cloning, there is a risk of an accumulation of deleterious recessive genes and mutations being introduced into the human genetic pool with an increase in various diseases and malformations.

Finally, cloning gives members of the present generation who put the procedure into practice a great deal of power in determining the genetic characteristics of future generations even though they will not be able to predict the nature of the future environment. Hence, the wrong people may be cloned for what the future demands. Moreover, there could be many social and political problems associated with the selection of people who would be given this power over man's genetic future.

Cloning could provide a solution to infertility in some situations. For example, it could be employed to allow women who cannot ovulate or who have no eggs, or men who have no sperm, to produce children of their own.[10] The male lacking sperm cells could arrange for a nucleus from one of his body cells to replace the nucleus of an egg cell from his wife. Similarly, the female without eggs could arrange for the nucleus of one of her body cells to replace the nucleus of an egg cell donated by another woman. The resulting embryo could then be transferred to the suitably prepared uterus of the nucleus donor or to that of the egg cell donor for further growth and development.

If one partner in a marriage had a severe hereditary defect, cloning with the other partner's genetic material would avoid the defect being transmitted to any offspring. Indeed, cloning may be necessary in future to complement sexual reproduction as part of any programme aimed at preventing deterioration of the human genetic pool.

In a somewhat more utilitarian vein, Fletcher[11] has proposed that clonees could act as organ donors for one another, thereby overcoming some of the present difficulties in obtaining vital organs for transplantation, for example, kidneys, and hearts. Fletcher also predicts that cloning will be necessary to produce people for special tasks in the community requiring special characteristics of a physical or mental nature. For example, he suggests that it would be an advantage to have people of smaller size for space flight since they would be better able to adapt to the conditions of space travel.

Probably one of the most important arguments in favour of cloning is that it will allow the study of factors responsible for cell growth, multiplication and differentiations.[12] This, in turn, may lead to a better understanding of and cure for cancer and infant malformations. Cloning would also allow the study of the ageing process in cells with the possibility of diminishing the rate of ageing and increasing the human lifespan. It could also lead to a better understanding of immunological responses of the body and thus have application to the management of allergies, infection, wound-healing and organ transplantation. Obviously, such studies would entail experimentation with the early embryo and might be opposed on the grounds of interference with human life and the possible production of abnormal embryos. In both situations, the embryos may have to be destroyed and again this would meet with strong moral objections by those who regard the early embryo as a definitive rather than a potential human being.

Ectogenesis
Ectogenesis is the term applied to growth of the embryo outside of the uterus. This occurs briefly during the procedure of IVF when after fertilization the very early embryo consisting of two cells is grown in a medium in the laboratory. In this chapter the term will be used to refer to the entire growth and development of the foetus outside of the uterine environment in the laboratory. This is not as far-fetched as it may sound because very small premature babies of less than 1000 g are already being kept alive in incubators in neonatal intensive care nurseries. Furthermore, they can survive and develop normally as far as can be determined in short-term follow-up studies. Although an artificial placenta has not yet been successfully designed

to support foetal life in the first half of pregnancy, the time is not far off when an embryo may be encouraged to grow and develop through foetal life to gestational maturity (thirty-seven to forty weeks).

Ectogenesis may allow women with various diseases to produce children. For example, women with poorly controlled drug-resistant high blood pressure in whom intrauterine pregnancy may cause a deterioration in their health or an increase in the height of the blood pressure, which in turn could lead to serious maternal and foetal complications, may be well advised to opt for ectogenesis rather than to attempt intrauterine pregnancy. Similarly, in those women who have had recurrent miscarriages in the first three months of pregnancy, where it has been established that the foetuses have been normal in development and where no obvious cause for the failure of the pregnancies has been found, ectogenesis may provide the solution to a barren marriage and the psychological trauma of repeated pregnancy loss.

Undoubtedly, ectogenesis would be necessary if the cloning of human beings was to go ahead enthusiastically in large numbers, since it would then be mandatory to have an environment in which to mature the embryos. If there were not enough uteri for this purpose, a suitable extrauterine environment would be essential or the embryos would have to be preserved by some method such as freezing. This would allow embryos to be kept until required or until a recipient uterus was available.

Furthermore, if frozen embryos were sent into space as a convenient means of transporting large numbers of our species compared with transportation of an equal number of adults, at their destination on another world, the embryos would need to be matured by ectogenesis for practical purposes.

Ethically, provided the procedure does not interfere with normal growth and development, the main objection to ectogenesis is that it would be so far removed from normal human nurturing that it would have a dehumanizing effect. The parent or parents, if there were any in the customary sense, would have much less contact with the foetus than in normal intrauterine pregnancy, and therefore both parents and child may show the adverse psychological effects of such separation. Moreover, there may be a loss of reverence for human life, as the foetus being matured by ectogenesis could come to be regarded by those in charge of the nurturing machinery as any other living thing rather than as a developing human being.

On the other hand, it could be argued that this speculation is fallacious in the light of the knowledge we have about parenting of premature babies, who may have to be cared for in incubators in the neonatal intensive care nursery for periods of three to four months continuously. In these circumstances the parents are encouraged to spend as much time as possible in the nursery with their baby and to identify closely with him or her. There is no evidence that parents or baby suffer adversely psychologically if close contact of this type is maintained throughout the baby's stay in the nursery.[13]

Another argument in support of ectogenesis is that total extrauterine development would eliminate maternal morbidity and mortality associated with intrauterine pregnancy and would obviate foetal birth trauma.[14] In addition, if the environment could be closely controlled without adverse side effects in the extrauterine situation, some foetal malformations caused by agents circulating in the mother, for example, drugs, including those used socially such as alcohol and tobacco and infective organisms, could be prevented altogether. In other words, it is conceivable that prospective parents may be able to protect their offspring better in a perfect artificial environment of ectogenesis than in the natural intrauterine one, exposed as it is to many adverse influences which cannot always be readily avoided in modern urban civilization.

A feminist view of childbirth is that it is barbaric, causing temporary deformation of the body, pain, and discomfort. Ectogenesis would spare women from the ordeal of pregnancy, labour, and delivery.[15]

Human-Animal Hybrids

In future it may be possible to insert human genetic material into an egg cell of an animal and so produce a man-animal hybrid. Initially, success is more likely to be achieved using egg cells of primates because of their closer relationship to humans on the evolutionary scale.

Edwards[16] probably echoes the sentiments of most of us when he states that such hybridization would be 'condemning the human component to a condition unworthy of it'. Leach[17] has also reminded biologists of the ancient Greek myth of the minotaur, which was a man-bull hybrid which was so dreadful to look upon that it had to be closed away in a labyrinth.

Fletcher[18] has put forward an alternative point of view, by suggesting that man-animal hybrids would be morally justified if they were able to protect human beings from danger, disease, or unpleasant occupations. Although they would be of lower intelligence than man, they would be able to carry out unpleasant jobs and mundane tasks in the community, relieving man for more skilled occupations.

It is not surprising that this topic more than any other engenders alarm, revulsion, and fear in most people. Biologists would be well advised to heed community opinion before starting any research of this nature, lest they provoke a serious backlash of considerable social, political, and legal proportions.

There seems little doubt that cloning and ectogenesis would allow the solution of some forms of human infertility and prevent some inherited and transmissible diseases. Probably more importantly, research associated with these techniques would lead to a better understanding and management of human cancer, ageing, and foetal malformations.

At the same time these techniques are open to serious ethical objections, and one would need to bear these in mind when reaching a decision about whether to proceed or not. If the decision is in the affirmative, appropriate ethical guidelines formulated by a body representing all interested parties should be observed.

Personally, I would endorse the opinion of Leroy Walters[19] who, after preparing an extensive survey of the ethical literature, concluded that 'laboratory *in vitro* fertilization research with early human embryos is in principle ethically acceptable, provided that the research seeks important information which cannot reasonably be acquired in any other way'.

Man-animal hybridization, however, is in a totally different category altogether, for reasons mentioned above, and should be eschewed completely unless a really convincing case can be made for its morality and its need.

12 With Child in Mind: The experience of a potential IVF mother

Isabel Bainbridge

To the Australian Aborigine the myths and legends of the dawning of time and of creation are told in the stories of the dreamtime. As dreamtime evolves it gives way to reality. Like all loved children, Stephen's existence began in dreamtime, and I want to share just a small part of his dreamtime with you.

In the days before IVF and long before I knew Toby, I knew and began to love my first child Stephen. I chose that name for him when I was fourteen. At twenty-one I married, and the time was ready for me to conceive my long-awaited and already loved baby.

While I waited for the first signs of pregnancy, Stephen slowly formed and devolped as part of my expected fertility. Stephen grew and kicked inside me; he kicked for life to begin. Outside him I planned his life. I made the clothes he would wear, chose the toys that would be a vital part of his development, read books on how to be a good mother, and talked about him with my friends.

Stephen's birth day was 6 August. He was born by normal delivery and at birth a wet, wrinkled baby was laid across my tummy. I felt his sodden dimpled hands grasping my fingers while his wet lips which touched my skin searched for food. His big, black, vacant eyes searched the room blindly. His puzzled expression pointed to his confusion as lights and noise and movement all jumbled in on his new existence.

Stephen weighed 4000 grams and had a crop of dark brown hair which fringed his pretty face. He had perfect skin and cherubic lips and large dark eyes which looked full of intelligence and gazed around to see where his next meal was coming from. Stephen's father played a loving and vital part in the conception and the birth day. He helped me magnificently through labour, and our relationship strengthened because of it. He played an important part in socializing Stephen. The father was to show the son what the world was all about and how to play the game.

Although we never spoke of it much, we both knew that Stephen was part of our growth towards maturity. The extra responsibility would cause us to extend ourselves, and to have more to give to the world and people around us. Life would develop for us because of Stephen. He would give as reasons to join in the celebration rituals which our family practices as relief from the daily struggle. As an adult, Stephen would play an important part in helping the world become a better place. Where we fail, he would conquer.

This is a small part of Stephen's dreamtime. There is so much more I could tell you, but that will have to wait for another time.

Stephen is a magic child; the dreamtime baby who has helped Toby and me to mature the way we have. He has been the cause of our disillusionment. He forced us into compromising situations. He made us change our attitudes and find happiness where we least expected it. He opened doors to new worlds. Because of Stephen we learned to make the best of life and to realize some of its many unexpected limitations. He taught us about faith and hope, about love and understanding.

You must be wondering what Stephen has to do with IVF!

Stephen is the child I have been attempting to conceive for the past seventeen years. Stephen is why Toby and I are involved in the IVF programme. Stephen is waiting inside my mind. His spirit lives inside me and waits for nature or my doctors to form his body — the body which will set him free to live. Only once in all my years as a midwife, I held a baby girl in my arms; she was the exact image of Stephen. So in real life I have held my dreamtime child in my arms, touched him, fed him, and looked after him. I know him. He began in me.

Stephen is one of the most deformed babies you will ever hear about. He has a handicap. He has no body. He has existed for a long time, waiting for his physical body to begin inside me — the body he will use as a vehicle to give quality to his existence.

Every creation starts with thoughts, ideas, and fantasy evolving into reality. Stephen lives in my mind just as part of every child lives in its mother's mind. Because of his deformity and my deformity,

I have kept him to myself. I am ashamed of him and of my infertility which keeps him from life. I am disgusted at the damage we have caused to each other's bodies. I want him to be separate and to begin to be responsible for his own life. I want to show him to the world and to be proud of him as I was in my teens before the accident of infertility occurred.

It is strange to let Stephen out. Perhaps I am brave enough to share part of the reality of my child with you because I want you to understand a little of why there is a need for the IVF programme and where it fails as the ultimate in treatment for infertility.

Stephen's story started somewhere in my childhood when I began to realize I would have a child one day. Later on the seed began to take shape, and at the age of fourteen I named him, and the seed started to grow roots.

In my late teens various episodes of a 'grumbling' appendix were considered to be a student nurse's excuse to get out of work. My complaints of pain were ignored until an ovarian cyst ruptured and a laparotomy proved that I also had a chronically inflamed appendix. That was in 1963. I learnt a few weeks ago, in 1981, that a 'grumbling' appendix is a major cause of tubal damage in girls and women of all ages in Australia. If only more general practitioners knew that and would act more promptly!

When I was twenty-one I started my attempt at pregnancy and began to realize that things were not going to be easy. Eventually, I had five years of very painful investigations and tubal treatments. The two major operations to repair my damaged Fallopian tubes only resulted in two ectopic pregnancies. Further repair work on what was left of my remaining tube was a waste of time. All my treatments were at considerable cost to myself and the community. The various gynaecologists I attended never mentioned the word infertility. They were there to help me achieve a pregnancy. My damaged tubes were the problem to be overcome. How can I recognize the word 'infertility' when my child is always there, waiting, ghostlike? He is like an actor in the wings waiting for his scene, waiting to play his part.

I have forgotten him at times. But he always reminds me that he is there. At times, the pain of Stephen kicking inside me emerged in the form of an acute anxiety state. I was treated as a neurotic woman and given sedative drugs rather than as an infertile woman who needed some pretty solid emotional support. Stephen and I are the survivors of a tragedy in which I lost my fertility and the body of my child. His deformed state is part of the quality of my life. What quality of life can I give him? Surely quality of life, like happiness, is something we each have to find for ourselves. It's not something I can force into another person's life, yet if I improve the quality of my own life it may benefit another life. The only way I can give quality to my child's life now is by giving him a body through which he can live. The only alternative is to destroy him. Who can help this mother practise euthanasia on her deformed child? How do you destroy a child with no body? How can you bury a child who hasn't known life, who is held back from any attempt at realizing his life because of his mother's deformity?

Toby and I have been involved with the IVF programme in Melbourne since 1978. We have had many discussions about what we are doing and why. We are part of the first generation of people who cannot turn to adoption for the easy answer to our problem. Recent publicity has made us stop and think. Are we doing the right thing by ourselves, our child, and our society?

On the question of there being far too many people in the world already, we can only say that Australia does not have that problem. We fail to see how it would help the world if we remain childless because other people cannot control their fertility. Surely it would be better that our child reaped the benefit of the accident of birth in Australia. If he was well educated by people who loved him dearly, he could help the world better than we can. We don't ignore the problem of overpopulation in other countries; it worries us too. We continue to live with the problem because there is nowhere else to go.

Other questions were raised such as, is it right for us to want a child when my body would no longer be able to conceive children naturally? Since we have always felt particularly fertile and have always wanted our child, we have always considered that we had as much right to choose children as any of our more fertile friends. In some respects our child has already chosen us. You don't suddenly stop wanting a child simply because of the physical problem. If you suddenly became blind in an accident, would you turn to your children and say, 'We don't want you now because we cannot see you'? It's the same for couples with an infertility problem. Because we can't see our children it doesn't stop them being there. Like blind parents we can still feel our child's presence. If we cannot make the body he requires, we will have done the best we can, and all three of us will have to live with that change of circumstance and make sure life improves despite problems. Assuming we are fully informed by our specialist, we have the same rights as any other person with a genuine human problem to seek ways of overcoming that problem.

I also had to ask the question, was it right to inflict so much treatment on myself? So far the IVF treatment, although emotionally exhausting at times, is the least physically invasive infertility treatment I've ever had. It is a tremendous worry to me these days to know that I have had at least twenty general anaesthetics and four major abdominal operations. Sometimes I feel I don't ever want to be touched surgically again. I feel I have lost my privacy. I see daily the effects that Stephen has already had on my body. IVF is my last attempt at pregnancy. It is the way that I shall keep my sanity through my menopause and later in my life. I will always know that I did the best I could. There is no other way to go for me, and I am lucky that Toby is happy to support me.

We also began to wonder if we had a right to be attempting treatment at cost to our community. After all, our problem is only one of many of the problems of our society. Compared to the cost of other treatment we have had, IVF will represent a very cost-effective treatment once it is out of the research stage. This treatment will help thousands in the future, and we feel we've repaid the price of our treatment by volunteering to take part in the research work, which is the only way this project can become available as a world-wide treatment for all who need it.

If I was protesting about the public cost of infertility treatments, I'd be 'up in arms' about the number of inexpert gynaecological operations performed every year by doctors who are not specialists in this field. They cause untold damage to infertile couples and create untold community expense, not necessarily because they are ignorant of the surgical techniques but mostly because they simply do not understand what infertility is all about. There is so much new knowledge and so many new techniques that can safely help the infertile couple these days that it seems strange that people opt for old-fashioned, painful, and damaging treatment from doctors who are sometimes obstetricians and gynaecologists but are not infertility specialists.

People who complain about the cost of infertility research and the IVF programme should examine the cost to the community of the long-term untreated unhappiness associated with infertility. The cost cannot be counted financially. In the long term the most cost-effective treatments will be reasonably safe and quick and cheap to perform while leaving minimal physical damage to the patient. IVF and artificial insemination both seem to meet these requirements. Yet governments still prefer to spend public money by funding the some-times more expensive, more dangerous, less successful major opera-tions as treatments for infertility.

No infertility treatment will be totally cost-effective unless some type of emotional counselling is offered concurrently with treatment. We have never been offered counselling as part of our infertility treatment. It would have helped. There were times in my twenties when I really thought that I was going crazy. Recently a gynaecologist mentioned in passing conversation, 'You're the least of my worries. You're one of my most well patients.' I wonder what he will think when he reads of Stephen. Even 'sensible me' has times when the mental anguish is hard to cope with and my stomach is held 'in a vice'. The few attempts at counselling that I chose when I really felt the need have not been part of my medical treatment. They helped in strange ways but I think they would have been far more effective if they had been directly linked with my treatment. I do not think that this is an area that the gynaecologist should take on as invariably he will not have sufficient time. Some type of counselling is even more urgently needed within the IVF programme because the treat-ment is not only far more emotionally exhausting than other infertility treatments, but for most couples in the programme it is 'the end of the road'. If it doesn't work for them, they simply have to face their infertility. For those who have never had any form of counselling and have not faced their infertility before, it can be devastating.

I am lucky to be able to talk about Stephen with you. It was frightening at first, but it has turned into quite a day's outing for him. We shall all sleep well tonight. I have met couples who keep their children locked away for a lifetime. They cannot talk for fear of misunderstanding or disbelief from their families and their com-munity, for fear of being treated as heretics.

The only way professionals can help people on the IVF programme to achieve their full potential is to allow us to take risks. To do this we need as much education as we can get while we are having our IVF treatment. We want to learn about the physical and emotional events that are happening to us. We want to make responsible decisions about our treatment. We have lost control of our fertility for so long now that we want to be the ones to have the responsibility of making the decisions at last. Recent media coverage would have the world believe that scientists and doctors invented IVF for their own amusement and that they are miracle workers who have taken over God's work. In fact, the entire programme started with infertile couples asking the doctors and scientists to help solve a problem. The miracle of life is that so many couples have braved the worst emotional storms and are still fighting. Maybe God could see we have a problem and nature wasn't being very helpful, so He planned that man should take over nature's job.

Scientists should not have to make ultimate ethical decisions regarding the morality of the work they do. If they have that power, people will sit back and let them use it. Likewise politicians and lawyers should not have the power of making the final judgement. It is ordinary people like us with intelligence and education who must use that power and tell the scientists how to help us and why we want to be helped. We must make the final decisions concerning the morality of what we are doing. We are the people who are shaping society and we must look to the good and the harm IVF can do to us. We must be responsible for our own destiny in making the world a better place in which to live for all of us at whichever level of society we choose to live.

Recently the human egg has caused a lot of concern. Should it be removed from the body to be fertilized, frozen, experimented on, and sometimes destroyed? It seems amazing that Australia has an army, navy, and airforce comprising men all happy to fight and maybe die for this country and a cause (that of securing freedom and dignity for those that live), yet some people are worried that human eggs should not die for an equally good cause. In each ovary there are hundreds of eggs which die in various stages of development in a woman's lifetime. Every month nature causes eggs, embryos, and sperm to die in random fashion. My eggs are merely the cells my ovaries produce. They are of no earthy use to me at present and will never form a foetus. If I had my ovaries totally removed no one would 'turn a hair', but because I have a couple of eggs removed, to be fertilized safe from the harm my body does them, it 'turns many heads'. I am happy if my doctors pick up an egg or two more than required. It's usual for some of the eggs not to become fertilized. I'd like to have the chance of having one or two put back. The excess fertilized eggs will be frozen for use in the next few months. I don't want my eggs to be kept for longer than a year or two. This will give me a second chance. If I have twins this time, I want my frozen eggs to be donated as soon as possible for use by another couple. I don't need to know the couple, but the eggs must be used soon. I don't really want them sitting around for hundreds of years. I'm not here to benefit a society hundreds of years hence. I'm here to benefit the society I live in now. I'd be very happy to donate my spare eggs to other couples, and I would relinquish all ownership of the eggs. If they could not be used for any reason it would be all right for them to be thrown away as long as I was informed. It's not that I don't value human life, but that I value a more mature form of existence. I don't think the human egg is the 'be all' and 'end all' of human existence, however much a miracle the new life is. If nature thought it more worthy of total protection then so would I.

IVF is merely part of today's changing world. We don't know yet the full reason for needing this knowledge. All I know is that we may need it desperately and urgently in the future if some virus or pesticide or other catastrophe happens. It will be of little use then for us to have to spend twenty or thirty years in research. IVF is merely a step in the evolving world, as anaesthesia was in the last century. At that time someone was supposed to have protested at the new outrage of the use of anaesthesia saying, 'Pain is an essential part of an operation — it is important for good recovery that the patient feels pain.' IVF is not the ultimate in treatments for infertility, only part of the miracle of the changing world we live in.

Everyone reacts to change according to his circumstances. Theologians, lawyers, and doctors are in the group of people who have been able to make easy choices about children. Mostly the fertile years are behind them. They have the time and money to be able to enjoy the luxury of debate — of thinking of imponderables. There is no urgent need for them to make decisions.

The couples who need to make choices about their fertility now are getting on with the job. They have no time to sit and think, 'Is IVF the right way to go?' For many, the only question they have ever asked is 'Do we want a baby?' They are now being asked to make decisions that their parents and grandparents never even thought about.

The law is on strange new territory with IVF, and personally, I am anxious about what it may do to the programme. An eminent lawyer said recently, 'We must stop the programme for a few years and consider the legal aspects.' I have the wierd feeling that the law is waiting until someone does something wrong, then it will legislate to make sure we don't make the same mistake again. Society is changing and this way of evolving laws is a stilted way of aiming at a better world. Surely the best way to keep the IVF programme safe is to have committees consisting of all manner of folk who are interested in the well-being of the programme. These committees will make sure that people can live up to the best values of the programme. IVF must only be used for the good of mankind as a whole. The decisions that these committees will make should become the law.

IVF techniques are a gift to the people and a safeguard that will ensure our future. The only way it will stay safe is by the education of infertile couples, professionals, and the community. Let's hope that Australia can show the world how to use this important work in a responsible way so that IVF only ever leads to the dignity of man and never to his destruction.

I could not have written this chapter without the special support of my husband, Toby. He has proved to be a good audience, editor, critic, and counsellor.

13 Conclusions — and Costs

William A. W. Walters and *Peter Singer*

This book covers a range of topics from diverse points of view. Looking over the articles we have commissioned, we thought it would be useful briefly to recapitulate the major themes. This final chapter is in one sense a summary of what has gone before. All the same, to call it a summary could be misleading for where our own ethical views differ from those of our contributors we have not hesitated to state our own positions. Of course, this gives us a final say. Our contributors have not had the opportunity to reply and you may wonder if this is an ethical way to treat them, but if this book is ever to appear the debate must stop somewhere.

The Moral Status of the Embryo

The most vehement opposition to the test-tube baby programme comes from those who believe that as soon as the egg and sperm have been united a new human being has come into existence. Those who hold this view of the starting point of human life then use it to reject IVF on the grounds that it is, at best, experimenting on human beings without their consent, and at worst, when it involves the disposal of embryos which for one reason or another cannot be re-implanted, the taking of innocent human life.

In his contribution to this book, Brian Johnstone describes some of the grounds on which it has been held that the embryo is entitled to the same kind of respect as a mature person. He refers to the biological continuity between embryo and adult and the difficulty in drawing a non-arbitrary line between the two. The argument is, in effect, that since there is no point at which we can say that the embryo *becomes* a person, we should hold that right from the start the embryo already *is* a person.

An alternative argument is based on the potential of the embryo to become a person. Even if the embryo is not yet an actual person, there is a high probability that in the normal course of its development it will become a person. Destroying the embryo therefore shows a reckless disregard for human life, akin to the recklessness that would be shown by a hunter shooting at a movement in some bushes when there was a high probability that the movement was that of a human being.

Against the first of these arguments one must place the obvious fact that the embryo involved in this research work consists of no more than a few cells. As Helga Kuhse and Peter Singer point out, the early embryo has none of the characteristics that we may normally think of as making human life worthy of respect and preservation. At this stage of its life, the embryo could not possibly even be sentient. So there are lines that can be drawn, in a non-arbitrary manner, between the early embryo and the mature human being. They may be 'fuzzy lines' in that the exact point at which, say, consciousness develops is difficult or even impossible to establish. But that is not a crucial objection. The fact that it is difficult to draw a sharp line between men who are bald and men who are not bald does not force us to say that a man with a smooth and shiny scalp is not bald, or that someone with a thick growth of hair is. When it comes to making practical decisions based on a fuzzy line of demarcation, we can always make sure that an error we may make is on the side of caution. Even so, there are cases about which there can be no doubt. That the embryo in the first day or two of its development is not sentient is beyond doubt.

The second argument, based on potential, must meet the objection that merely keeping egg and sperm apart also prevents a human life from coming into existence. This point has received sufficient discussion in the essay by Kuhse and Singer and needs no recapitulation here. It suffices to say that in our view the IVF programme is one which creates the possibility of human life where before there was none. To object to it on the grounds that it destroys potential human life is to apply a 'pro-life' principle in such a way as to bring about consequences which are in diametric opposition to the spirit of the principle itself.

We therefore conclude that arguments based on the moral status of the embryo do not present any conclusive objections to IVF. For similar reasons, if in order to improve the prospects of successful fertilization it is necessary to produce more embryos than can be re-implanted into the woman seeking to become pregnant, we believe this to be ethically acceptable. We believe that any excess embryos produced may either be preserved by freezing or disposed of, in accordance with the preferences of the biological parents.

Consent

As Brian Carey has said in his chapter on the problem of informed consent, most people agree that it is wrong to experiment on human beings unless the subjects of the experiment have given their consent, based on adequate information about the risks involved in taking part in the research. Where a person is incapable of giving informed consent, perhaps because of youth or mental defect, informed consent is generally obtained from a parent or guardian.

No one denies that for research into IVF to be ethical, the researchers must first have the informed consent of the woman who supplies the egg and the man who supplies the sperm. There is usually no problem about obtaining this, since the procedure offers the couple hope of having a much-wanted child. Nor does the procedure involve much risk to the mother. If it were proposed to attempt to transfer the embryo into a 'surrogate' mother, rather than into the woman from whom the egg was obtained, there would be a third party whose consent would need to be obtained; but again, since the surrogate mother would enter into the arrangement voluntarily, there should be no difficulty about obtaining informed consent.

The real ethical issue about consent in this kind of research relates to the embryo and the future individual it will become. Obviously it is not possible to obtain the consent of the embryo, still less of the individual the embryo will become. Does this make the research unethical?

Focussing for the moment on the embryo, we would hold, in line with what we have already said about the moral status of the embryo, that the embryo does not count as a person and hence that there is no objection to experimenting on it without its consent. In the case of purely experimental work, say on a 'surplus' embryo, it would seem right to obtain the consent of the parents, but this would not be proxy consent on behalf of the embryo. It would, instead, be the consent of the parents for a particular use to be made of something that they may still regard as their own biological material.

Should it ever prove possible to grow an embryo outside a human body, not just for a day or two but for several weeks, it would become necessary to re-examine this issue. If there is a possibility of the embryo being conscious, the ethics of performing an experiment on it are very different from when consciousness is out of the question.

Finally, what of the future individual who will be produced if the procedure of IVF and ET is successful? This future individual will become a mature human being. Will this human being have been the subject of an experiment that took place without his or her consent? That seems to be the case, at least as long as the procedure is regarded as experimental. In some respects that time has already passed, for several normal babies have been produced and the surgical techniques are now almost routine. On the other hand it must be admitted that no test-tube baby is yet old enough for his or her intellectual development to have been observed during the school years; nor are there yet enough test-tube babies for anyone to be able to state with confidence that the incidence of birth defects is no greater than normal. We are not suggesting, of course, that there is any good reason why the intellectual development of test-tube babies should be anything other than normal, or the incidence of birth defects greater. The point is only that the procedure may still be regarded as experimental because of the absence of this kind of evidence.

If the procedure is experimental in this sense, is it wrong because of the absence of consent from the individual to be created? We believe that in this situation it is legitimate to ask: will the individual be glad that the procedure was performed, when he or she is old enough to understand the question? Since the individual would not even have existed had the procedure not been performed, and since there is nothing to suggest that the lives of test-tube babies will be so miserable that they will regret being alive, it seems clear that the individuals will be glad that the procedure that made their lives possible was performed. In this sense they will give retrospective informed consent to what was done.

We would not suggest that retrospective informed consent is always an acceptable substitute for actual informed consent at the time of the experiment. In the special circumstance of the case we are considering, however, we would regard the probability of such retrospective consent as sufficient justification for going ahead. After all, those who hold that the procedure should not go ahead in the absence of actual consent by the future individual are saying that such procedures should not go ahead at all. Is this better for those who may have been created? Although it is true that those who would stop the procedure will never be blamed by those beings whose existence their position would prevent, it is also true that only those who take a more positive view will be able to receive the thanks of those whose existence their view has made possible.

Sexual Ethics

What does IVF have to do with sexual ethics? As both Helga Kuhse and William Daniel have pointed out, IVF completes the separation between sex and reproduction that began when effective contraceptives became available. Now we can have sex without having children, and children without having sex. Why, then, should one bring up questions of sexual ethics in connection with a technique which consists precisely in avoiding the sexual element of more commonplace reproduction?

William Daniel examines some of the aspects of sexual ethics that have been brought up in connection with IVF. There is, for instance, the fact that the normal way to obtain the sperm is by masturbation. According to some traditional views, masturbation is wrong. Daniel points out, however, that the chief reason for holding masturbation to be wrong — that it directs sexuality inwards to oneself, rather than outwards to another person — does not apply when the whole point of the act is to procreate. So the part played by masturbation in the creation of a test-tube baby does not seem to be a serious objection.

Daniel is more concerned about the effect that separating love and procreation will have on marriage. The intrusion of technology into the act of procreation carries with it, he believes, the threat of a devaluation of sexual intimacy and ultimately the prospect of grave assaults on marriage and the family. Nevertheless, where a husband and wife cannot have the child they desire through normal sexual means, Daniel accepts that IVF will not be untrue to their relationship.

Surely no one who has read Isabel Bainbridge's contribution to this book could disagree with Daniel on that; but we would go further. Daniel explicitly limits his acceptance of IVF to married couples. We would agree that IVF should only be offered in situations in which any child that may be born would have the best possible prospects of a good start in life. The scarcity of the medical rescources needed for IVF is enough reason to see that their use is limited in this manner. We cannot, however, endorse the assumption that only legally married couples can provide a child with a good home environment. We can imagine other evidence of a sound relationship between people who, for one reason or another, are not married. We do not believe that there is any moral principle that would rule out IVF where such evidence is available.

The Family

If IVF can strengthen, rather than weaken, the relationship between a couple, are there any grounds for concern about the effect it may have on the family as a whole? John Henley finds such grounds in the necessity for screening couples who are to be offered treatment, and also that support groups have been established for couples involved in the programme. Both points suggest that there is stress and frustration involved in the process. To be refused treatment must be a bitter disappointment; and to undergo treatment that proves unsuccessful could be even more depressing.

It would be wrong to deny the substance of these points. We should be aware that the decision to offer IVF will have among its consequences some unhappiness on the part of those who seek help from the programme but cannot be helped. Yet to use this as a basis for rejecting IVF is to adopt a paternalistic attitude to those who wish to try to have a child by this method. If couples are fully informed, both of the possibility of rejection, and of the possibility of the treatment turning out to be unsuccessful, should not the final choice be up to them? To say that we should not offer them the choice of treatment is to say that we are in a better position than they are to judge what they should be prepared to risk in order to have a child.

We would question this degree of paternalism in this situation. In his classic work *On Liberty*, John Stuart Mill argued that people are normally the best judges of their own interests. As long as they are fully informed, people should not be prevented from undertaking a risky act (Mill's example was crossing an unsafe bridge) because 'no one but the person himself can judge of the sufficiency of the motive which may prompt him to incur the risk'. There may be exceptions to Mill's rule, but in our view IVF is not one of them. One would have to be bold, or foolish, to be sure that the possibility of having a child does not, for a given couple, outweigh the risks of rejection and failure involved in applying for IVF.

As for other effects on the family, we do not see any problems arising from IVF followed by ET to the womb of the egg donor. If the sperm used was that of the legal or de facto husband the child would be as completely a child of that couple as any child produced by more common means. Where the sperm is that of a donor who is not the husband, the situation is parallel to that of children produced through AID. As John Morgan points out in his chapter, there is no evidence that family life for children conceived through AID is any worse than family life for other children. So here, too, there is little basis for particular concern about the effects of IVF on family life. One could argue that children born through this method have better prospects for a good family life than normal children, because they will all be children that their parents very much wanted to have.

Should the fertilized embryo be transferred into a woman who is not the genetic mother, different problems may arise. We discuss these under the heading 'surrogate mothers'.

The Cost

When all the specific objections to aspects of IVF have been discussed, there is still one troubling question that hangs over the entire issue: is it worth the expense? Medical resources are limited. To give money to one area of medicine is to withhold money from another. If our medical spending is to be rational rather than haphazard, we should make some attempt to sort out our priorities. In doing so, where should we place IVF?

In discussing this question, it will be useful to distinguish two possible perspectives from which it may be asked. On the one hand, one could ask, 'If we were to distribute in a perfectly rational manner all the resources we now spend on medicine, would we still be allocating resources to test-tube baby research?' Alternatively, one could ask, 'Given the present overall situation with regard to the distribution of medical resources, is there anything particularly inappropriate about the amount we are spending on test-tube baby research?'

The first of these perspectives attempts to measure the amount we spend on test-tube babies against some ideal standard; the second measures it against the standard of our current pattern of expenditure. Obviously these are very different standards. In an ideal world, each dollar of medical expenditure would be used to maximum effect to eliminate illness and disability wherever it occurs. Thus we would not have a situation in which millions of children die from malnutrition (and from the diseases that afflict the malnourished because they are too weak to resist) while major hospitals develop coronary care units that are marvels of technology but of uncertain value in saving lives. There can be little doubt that more lives would be saved by providing adequate food and a very basic level of health care for those who need it than by providing the latest electronic equipment for heart attack victims. This kind of redistribution, however, would require the wealthy nations to share more equally with the poorer nations, and this is something that the wealthy nations have so far been unwilling to do.

Even if we limit our attention to a single nation such as Australia, similar irrationalities in the use of medical resources are not hard to find. Once again, the large sums spent on the most sophisticated forms of intensive care would be difficult to justify when compared with the relatively small amounts required to make real inroads into infant mortality, blindness, and infectious disease among Aborigines.

We may lament this situation, we may — we should — try to change it; but we would be unrealistic if we did not acknowledge that there are powerful institutional barriers to an ideally rational ordering of medical expenditure. Those in leading positions in politics, the media, the civil service, and the medical establishment can be expected to have a built-in bias towards more resources for the kind of conditions from which they, their families, and their friends are likely to suffer, and these conditions include heart attacks but not malnutrition-related diseases. Moreover, doctors and medical researchers themselves are naturally attracted towards those areas of research and treatment that present the most interesting challenges to their intellect and skill. These are not necessarily the areas that offer the greatest benefits to patients per dollar spent.

Hence to measure the justifiability of spending on test-tube baby research against an ideally rational scale of priorities is to apply a standard so exacting that it would condemn a good deal of widely accepted medical expenditure. If we are considering the ethics of test-tube baby research in particular, rather than undertaking a general assessment of all medical expenditure, perhaps this is an unduly stringent standard to apply.

Measured against the standard of our current pattern of expenditure, test-tube baby research does not look so bad. Although it is true that infertility is not a life-threatening condition, it is impossible to read the chapter Isabel Bainbridge has written for this book without under-standing what a distressing condition it can be. Jan Brennan, the mother of a test-tube baby, described herself as a person with a disability or handicap. That seems a proper way of describing in-fertility. There is something normal women can do that an infertile woman cannot do. Some infertile women may not have a strong desire to have children, and in that case their disability does not trouble them; but others obviously find their disability a major threat to their happiness. The use of medical resources, within limits, to help them overcome the disability seems perfectly appropriate.

If it is proper to spend some money to help the infertile, the only question about the allocation of resources in this area is whether more money is being spent than can be justified. Here we have to distinguish between the costs of the treatment and the costs of the research that made the treatment possible. By far the largest costs were the research costs. The treatment has now reached the point where it can be regarded as almost routine, even though the success rate is still low, and it is not a particularly expensive form of treatment when compared with the costs of other medical procedures.

The research that went into making IVF possible was expensive: the Melbourne team received roughly $1 million in assistance from various sources. But even this sum is not a vast amount by the standards of medical research expenditure, and it has, unlike a lot of medical research, produced both new knowledge and practical results. The new knowledge could have application to areas other than overcoming infertility. For instance, understanding how fertil-ization occurs also involves understanding what prevents fertilization. Thus new and better methods of contraception, perhaps even a male contraceptive, may emerge from this research. That could be a spin-off that would change the attitudes of those who object to test-tube babies because of the world population problem. It would, moreover, be a spin-off that made the original research highly cost-effective.

Paying for medical research is always a gamble, because results can never be guaranteed in advance. Some people would say that you should not even ask for a likelihood of useful results, since an addition to basic knowledge is as much as can be hoped for, and basic knowledge may always prove at some future time to have useful applications that we could never have foreseen. The money spent on IVF research could be defended in this way, but it does not have to be, for it is a piece of research that has been remarkably successful in producing both new knowledge and immediate practical applications. As such it appears to have given an unusually good return for the money it required.

The Created Individual

John Morgan devotes the major part of his chapter to a discussion of the ethical arguments for and against artificial (laboratory) human reproduction versus normal coital reproduction. He concludes that 'the integrity of the procreative process is not attacked by IVF where the embryo conceived is the expression and embodiment of love, since the child is the result of a decision from within the procreative context of hubsand and wife'. We agree entirely with him when he writes further, 'at this point technology is simply being used in the service of humanity and need not threaten or diminish it, unless we exchange an ethic of responsibility for one of irresponsibility in our exercise of creativity'.

From the created individual's point of view, concern has been expressed that IVF and ET could result in an increased number of foetal abnormalities and that for this reason alone the procedures should be abandoned. Although the answer to this question is not yet known, because of the small number of babies conceived by this method, animal studies have not shown any significant increase in foetal abnormalities as a result of IVF. Hence this is not likely to become an important consideration.

Probably one of the most important aspects of IVF and ET is that concerning the effect of the nature of the conception on the created individuals in later life. Will the individuals suffer psychlogically and emotionally because of the nature of their conception? Will they lack a sense of uniquesness or self? Will they become anti-social misfits? Again we have no conclusive answers to such questions, but anecdotal evidence suggests that children conceived by AID, who may be regarded as an analagous group, do not have any greater difficulties in society than those conceived normally. Furthermore, as the children conceived by IVF are brought into a loving and caring environment, it is much more likely that they will be better adjusted in the wider society than the unfortunate children conceived normally and born unwanted into an undesirable emotional environment.

As long as IVF and ET are used to solve human infertility problems and are controlled adequately so that they are not used indiscriminately for experimental purposes, we see them as a positive step in relieving the suffering of infertility and maintaining the stability of marriage. Further, we see no valid reason for supposing that the individual created by IVF should be at any greater disadvantage in later life after birth than any other member of society conceived in the usual way.

Surrogate Motherhood

As Alan Rassaby points out in Chapter 10 of this book, although surrogate motherhood is frequently thought about and referred to in relation to recent advances in human reproductive biology, it has been practised since biblical times. We know of recent cases in our community where the arrangements for surrogate motherhood have been made privately among the people concerned including medical practitioners and solicitors. Usually, the procedure is a last resort for an infertile couple whose desire for a child cannot be met for various reasons by any other means, including adoption and IVF. This being the case, the infertile couple see surrogacy as an arranged adoption. The surrogate, on the other hand, sees her role as one of demonstrating compassion or providing a service for financial reward.

Although it can be argued that surrogacy should be proscribed because it is morally unacceptable, this would seem to deny other similar acts already widely used and accepted by society such as blood, tissue and organ donations, wet-nursing, and AID.

The objections to surrogacy based on fears of financial exploitation of the surrogate and the person who seeks her services are very real and must be taken seriously, but government regulations could be made to protect both people from exploitation. They could also provide for privacy, confidentiality, medical insurance to cover complications of pregnancy in the surrogate, and contractual arrangements. Although there is a possibility that a woman may be coerced into the surrogate role if she is below the poverty line and unemployed, she may prefer to make money by this means than by other perhaps less fulfilling activities, such as monotonous factory labour or even prostitution.

The dangers of emotional trauma to the mother bearing the child when she has to pass it over to the would-be parents if she does not want to give up the baby at birth are also formidable. It may be possible to ease these dangers by adequate counselling, which would aim to eliminate potential surrogates who are likely to experience such trauma most severely. At this stage we have insufficient experience to say how serious this problem will turn out to be. Obviously any surrogacy programme would need to begin cautiously and to keep a close watch on this problem.

One of the most difficult problems that may arise is that of foetal abnormality. Would the prospective parents be emotionally capable of accepting an abnormal baby if this unfortunately occurred? To some extent antenatal intrauterine diagnosis tests in the early second trimester of pregnancy would enable some abnormalities to be diagnosed and the pregnancy to be terminated. But the majority of foetal abnormalities cannot be diagnosed at this early stage of pregnancy, and one may not know that the baby has an abnormality until it is home. This is not a risk peculiar to surrogacy, however; all pregnant women face similar risks, the magnitude of which depends on the circumstances of the particular case. For these reasons we would not find this a substantial enough argument to proscribe surrogacy. The prospective parents would have to accept the risk of foetal abnormality and assume responsibility for an abnoraml child in the same way that they would have to accept it if it had resulted from their own pregnancy, provided that the surrogate mother had not done anything during the course of the pregnancy that was known to increase the chance of foetal abnormality. Critics of surrogate motherhood often emphasize that the procedure is totally unacceptable because the child-to-be is unable to give consent to being born under such unusual circumstances and that the prospective parents are being indulged in their selfish desire to have a child by whatever means possible. The prospective parents, in other words, are putting their own interests before those of the child. But surely, in practice, all prospective parents have children in response to their desire for children rather than for any other motive. Hence in this respect, the surrogacy situation is much the same as is the normal one.

Whether the child born by a surrogate mother should have access to the precise circumstances of his origin is a contentious issue. We would argue that the child has this right and that he could exercise it beyond a particular age if he wished by consulting a Registry Office. The information given would be strictly confidential, and no details of the whereabouts of the surrogate mother would be given.

In our opinion, surrogate motherhood is ethically acceptable and similar to adoption. It can be viewed as an arranged adoption. Provided it is adequately controlled, as suggested by Rassaby, and used to help infertile couples in whom all other measures have failed or have minimal chance of success, we can see no convincing ethical reason for its proscription.

Cloning, Ectogenesis and Human-Animal Hybridization

Cloning of humans is not a practical proposition at present and even if it does become possible in the foreseeable future, it is difficult to see how it would ever have a prominent place in human reproduction. Although it may be thought to be advantageous to create 'carbon-copies' of individual genotypes, it would still require the passage of at least twenty to thirty years before such clonees could play a significant role in society. In that period the environment may have changed considerably, requiring people with different attributes from those of the previous generation. Alternatively, the environment may have so affected the physical, mental, and psychological development of the clonee that he would reach adult life being very different from his 'identical' parent.

Cloning may have a small place, however, in the avoidance of hereditary disorders where one partner in a marriage has or carries the disorder. Under such circumstances, the other healthy partner could reproduce by cloning, so avoiding the disease in the clonee.

Human reproduction aside, cloning may have an important role to play in the study of factors involved in cell growth and differentiation, and hence could be of great importance in our understanding of disturbances of growth and development such as in cancer, ageing and foetal malformations. This would involve experimentation with the early human embryo, which in our opinion is ethically acceptable if the information to be gained cannot be readily obtained in any other way, provided that the embryo is at an early stage of development before it can be regarded as a sentient being.

Ectogenesis, or the entire development of the foetus outside of the uterus, is also far from practical realization, but it may eventuate with the efflux of time as smaller and smaller preterm babies are being sustained in neonatal intensive care nurseries. Again, we do not see any convincing ethical objection to ectogenesis, provided that it is used to sustain life which may otherwise be lost as, for example, in the case of an extremely premature baby or in the case of a woman who has a disorder which makes pregnancy dangerous or unsuccessful.

Human-animal hybridization is fraught with so many serious ethical problems, as outlined by William Walters earlier in this book, that we see no reason for embarking on such a complex and hazardous exercise. As far as we can determine, the ethical balance is weighed heavily against hybridization.

Appendix 1
Public Opinion Polls

Peter Singer

In June 1981 the Roy Morgan Research Centre sought the opinions of a cross section of Australian men and women about IVF and ET. Their survey provides the only objective indication so far of the views of the Australian public on the issues discussed in this book. Earlier opinion polls had been taken in the United States. The purpose of this appendix is to present a summary of the results of the Australian poll, and compare it with the results obtained in the United States.

The Australian poll was based on a sample of 1002 people. They were first asked: 'Have you heard of the test-tube method for helping married couples who can't have children?' Ninety-nine per cent of all people surveyed said that they had heard of this method. They were then asked: 'Do you approve or disapprove of the test-tube baby method for helping married couples who can't have children?' By far the majority, 77 per cent, indicated that they approved. Only 11 per cent disapproved, the remaining 12 per cent being undecided.

People were asked to give reasons for their attitudes. The precise question was: 'Why especially do you feel that way?' Of those who approved of the method, the most popular reply (19 per cent) was that it gives people the opportunity to have children. Similar replies, referring to the difficulty of adoption and the lack of preferable alternatives, added up to another 23 per cent. Seven per cent said that the decision was up to the parents; 6 per cent simply said that they could see nothing wrong with the method.

Only 1.5 per cent of all respondents referred to their religious beliefs as the basis of their attitude. Just under 5 per cent objected to the method on the grounds that it is 'not natural'. Less than 1 per cent regarded it as a waste of money.

The people surveyed were then told that at present married couples who have test-tube baby treatment have to pay $350 per treatment, and that about one treatment in eight has been successful in producing a baby. They were then asked: 'In your opinion, should couples be able to claim their test-tube baby treatment on health insurance, or not?' The replies indicated that 70 per cent of the sample thought couples should be able to claim the treatment on health insurance, 21 per cent thought they should not, and 9 per cent were undecided.

A more detailed analysis of the responses shows that approval of the test-tube baby method was relatively evenly distributed across Australia, including both city and country areas. Slightly more women approved than men, but the difference was only 3 per cent. Among those over fifty years old, disapproval was notably higher, reaching a peak of 17.4 per cent among males over fifty. Approval tended to be higher among those with professional and managerial occupations, and among those with higher incomes. Religion also showed some correlation with attitudes to the test-tube baby method. Approval among Roman Catholics was, at 67 per cent, significantly lower than among the sample as a whole. It was similar among Baptists and lower still (61 per cent) among those who belonged to a non-Christian religion. Yet in all these groups a clear majority approved. Adherents of the Anglican, Presbyterian, and United Churches had a higher degree of approval than the sample as a whole. So did those who said they had no religion.

In the United States opinion surveys were made in August 1978 by both the Gallop and Harris organizations. Both were based on samples of approximately 1500 people, but while the Gallup poll included males and females, the Harris poll interviewed women only. Although at the time the polls were taken only one test-tube baby had been born, the Gallup poll found that 93 per cent of their sample had heard or read about the birth.

The polls showed that a clear majority of Americans approved of the method. Yet, at least in 1978, the verdict was not quite as overwhelmingly in favour as it was in Australia in 1981. The Gallup poll indicated that 60 per cent of all Americans approved of the method and 27 per cent were opposed to it, the remaining 13 per cent being undecided. The Harris poll gave rise to some curious findings: on a general question about 'approval of the procedure', only 52 per cent approved, with 24 per cent disapproving and an equal number undecided. Yet 85 per cent of the sample were prepared to agree that the procedure should be available to married couples who are otherwise unable to have children. This suggests that inclusion of the word 'married' and a reference to the inability to have children prompts a more favourable response than a general question about 'approval of the procedure'. This could, at least in part, explain why the Australian poll reported a higher favourable response than the American Gallup poll.

The Harris poll also asked some more specific questions which are related to some of the points raised in this book. Firstly, in contrast to the 85 per cent who accepted the procedure for married couples unable to have children, only 21 per cent thought it should be available to unmarried couples who are living together and unable to have children. This figure is a little *less* than the figure (22 per cent) of those who thought it should be available to single women who are unable to have children. (The difference is puzzling, but may reflect the idea that the unmarried couple are living in sin, whereas the test-tube method enables a single woman to have a child without having sexual intercourse.) Only 11 per cent thought that the procedure should be available to lesbians or homosexuals. (It is not clear what difference the addition of 'or homosexuals' was understood to make. Was it a reference to homosexual males? If so, was it envisaged that the homosexual would fertilize an embryo to be implanted in a surrogate mother who would surrender it to the male homosexual? It would obviously have been better to treat lesbians and male homosexuals separately, since lesbians would not require the use of a surrogate.)

More women than not, by 49 per cent to 40 per cent, believed that where the husband is unable to provide healthy sperm, a married couple should be allowed to use donor sperm.

Finally, those surveyed were asked if they would allow doctors to remove more than one egg from a woman, fertilize them all, and then discard all but the one to be inserted for development. Forty-five per cent said they would allow this, 40 per cent said they would not, and 14 per cent were unsure. Disapproval of the discarding of the fertilized eggs was higher, but still not overwhelming, among Catholics. Thirty-nine per cent of Catholics said they would allow the additional eggs to be discarded, 48 per cent said they would not, and 12 per cent were unsure.

Sources

Information on the Australian poll was kindly provided by the Roy Morgan Research Centre Pty Ltd, Melbourne. Results of the US polls are included in the Ethics Advisory Board report, *HEW Support of Research Involving Human In Vitro Fertilization and Embryo Transfer*, Washington, D.C., 4 May 1979, Appendix.

Appendix II Ethical Guidelines for Clinicians and Scientists involved in IVF and ET

1 In all procedures associated with in vitro fertilization and embryo transplantation the particular moral viewpoint of the parents should be respected even if this viewpoint happens to be at variance with that of the clinician or scientist concerned.

2 As the entire procedure of in vitro fertilization and embryo transplantation involves a series of steps occurring over a variable period of time, it is important that the parents should be informed that their consent to in vitro fertilization and embryo transplantation is such that they can withdraw at any stage.

3 In view of the publicity surrounding in vitro fertilization and embryo transplantation, it is important that the anonymity of the parents be preserved by the medical team. Should the parents wish publicity they should authorize it by signing the appropriate consent form.

4 It is realized that in vitro fertilization and embryo transplantation have so far only been used in situations where the parents are legally married. The possibility of using in vitro fertilization and embryo transplantation in de facto or other relationships raises a number of complex moral and legal problems which need to be explored in depth before the Ethics Committee could support such proposals.

5 As a freezing technique has now been developed to allow the development of the zygote to be temporarily suspended by freezing, it is recommended that this technique be used when the in vitro fertilization procedure has produced an excess of normal zygotes

and/or the present conditions for implantation are less than optimal. It is anticipated that implantation will take place as soon as conditions are considered optimal. Should abnormal zygotes be detected, it is recommended that they should be appropriately examined to find out the cause of the abnormality and thereby, hopefully, enable it to be prevented in the future.

6 Parents will give informed consent to any procedure that may be undertaken on the zygote.

7 Once the embryo has been implanted, should any foetal abnormality be detected, before any action is taken, the parents should be fully informed of the nature of any foetal abnormality so that they can make a decision concerning termination or continuation of the pregnancy.

8 In the present state of development of the relatively new techniques of in vitro fertilization and embryo transplantation, it is justifiable to select parents who have already had children as their reproductive systems have already been successfully tested, but it is recommended that when the procedures of in vitro fertilization and embryo transplantation have become well established the priority should favour those parents who have not yet had any children.

Reproduced by permission of the Board of Management of the Queen Victoria Medical Centre, Melbourne.

References

Chapter 1   IVF and ET

1 H. Leridon, *Human Fertility: The Basic Components*, University of Chicago Press, Chicago, 1977; and R. V. Short, 'When a Conception Fails to Become a Pregnancy', CIBA Foundation Symposium 64, *Maternal Recognition of Pregnancy*, Excerpta Medica, Amsterdam, 1979, pp. 377–94.

2 A. M. Siegler, 'Tubal Plastic Surgery, the Past, the Present, the Future, *Obstetric and Gynaecological Survey*, vol. 15, pp. 608–701.

3 R. M. L. Winston, 'Microsurgical Tubocornual Anastomosis for Reversal of Sterilisation', *Lancet*, vol. 1, 1977, pp. 284–5.

4 A. O. Trounson, J. F. Leeton, C. Wood, J. Webb, and J. Wood, 'Pregnancies in Humans by Fertilization In Vitro and Embryo Transfer in the Controlled Ovulatory Cycle', *Science*, vol. 212, 1981, pp. 681–2.

5 J. D. Biggers, 'In Vitro Fertilization and Embryo Transfer in Human Beings', *New England Journal of Medicine*, vol. 304, 1981, pp. 336–42.

6 P. Renou, A. O. Trounson, C. Wood, and J. F. Leeton, 'The Collection of Human Oocytes for In Vitro Fertilization. I. An Instrument for Maximizing Oocyte Recovery Rate', *Fertility and Sterility*, vol. 35, 1981, p. 409.

7 L. R. Mohr and A. O. Trounson, 'The Use of Fluorescein Diacetate to Assess Embryo Viability in the Mouse', *Journal of Reproduction and Fertility*, vol. 58, 1980, pp. 189–96.

8 C. Wood, A. O. Trounson, J. F. Leeton, J. McK. Talbot, B. Buttery, J. Webb, J. Wood, and D. Jessup, 'A Clinical Assessment of Nine Pregnancies Obtained by In Vitro Fertilization and Embryo Transfer', *Fertility and Sterility*, vol. 35, 1981, pp. 502–8.

9 CIBA Foundation 52, *The Freezing of Mammalian Embryos*, Elsevier, North Holland, 1977.

Chapter 3   An Ethical Approach to IVF and ET

1 This line is from John Donne's poem, *The First Anniversary*.
2 For an interpretation of the 'sanctity of life' concept in terms of a 'sacred process' see K. Baier, 'The Sanctity of Life', *Journal of Social Philosophy*, vol. 5, April 1974, pp. 1–4.
3 Editorial, *The Medical Journal of Australia*, vol. 1, 64th year, no. 24, 11 June 1977, p. 871.
4 B. A. Santamaria: 'Medics "play God" with Babes on Ice', *Perth Independent*, 26 May 1981.
5 Arthur Schopenhauer, *On the Basis of Morality*, trans. E. F. J. Payne, Bobbs-Merrill Co., Indianapolis, 1965, p. 39.
6 This view is put forward by the theologian E. J. Carnell, *An Introduction to Christian Apologetics*, Grand Rapids/Eerdmans Publishing Co., 1950, as cited by R. B. Brandt: *Ethical Theory*, Prentice Hall, Englewood Cliffs, 1959, p. 67.
7 Plato's argument against defining 'good' in terms of the will of gods is in his *Euthyphro* (various translations and editions). It is sometimes thought that the dilemma can be avoided because God is good and could hence not have loved, or willed, torture. But to suggest that God is good implies that there must, already, be standards of good and bad independent of the love of God.
8 W. G. Sumner, *Folkways*, Ginn and Company, Boston, 1934, pp. 418, 28, as cited by Brandt, *Ethical Theory*, p. 59.
9 The quotation is from E. Wilson, *Sociobiology, The New Synthesis*, Harvard University Press, Cambridge, Mass., 1975, p. 562; for an interpretation of the relationship between sociobiology and ethics see Peter Singer, *The Expanding Circle — Ethics and Sociobiology*, Farrar, Strauss & Giroux, New York, 1981.
10 Karl Marx, 'The German Ideology' in *Writings of the young Marx on Philosophy and Society*, ed. and trans. L. D. Easton and K. H. Gudat, Anchor Books, Garden City, 1967, p. 463.
11 C. L. Stevenson puts forward a defence of emotivism in his *Ethics and Language*, Yale University Press, New Haven, 1944; J. M. Urmson: *The Emotive Theory of Ethics*, Hutchinson, London, 1968, provides a critical assessment. R. M. Hare's prescriptivism is expounded in *The Language of Morals*, Oxford University Press, London, 1952; and in *Freedom and Reason*, Oxford University Press, London, 1963; J. L. Mackie, *Ethics: Inventing Right and Wrong*, Penguin Books, Harmondsworth, 1977, de-

fends a version of subjectivism; as does J. C. C. Smart in *Utilitarianism for and Against*, Cambridge University Press, Cambridge, 1973.

12 David Hume's 'Essay on Suicide' is reprinted in various editions; for example, in S. Gorovitz *et al.* (eds), *Moral Problems in Medicine*, Prentice Hall, Englewood Cliffs, 1976, pp. 381–7. The quotation appears on p. 384.

13 David Hume, *An Enquiry Concerning the Principles of Morals*, section IX, part I, various editions.

14 For the formulations of the universalizability see Immanuel Kant, *Groundwork of the Metaphysics of Morals*, trans. H. J. Paton, Hutchinson, London, 1976, p. 67; Hare, *Freedom and Reason*; J. Habermas, *Legitimation Crisis*, trans. T. McCarthy, Beacon Press, Boston, 1975, pp. 102–10. The quotation can be found on p. 108.

15 Mackie, *Ethics*, p. 123.

16 R. Veatch, 'The Ethics of Miracles' in *Newsweek*, 19 September 1977. My emphasis.

17 Habermas, *Legitimation Crisis*, p. 12.

18 Singer, *The Expanding Circle*, p. 143.

19 See, for example, M. Tooley, 'Abortion and Infanticide', *Philosophy and Public Affairs*, vol. 2, 1972; P. Singer, *Practical Ethics*, Cambridge University Press, Cambridge, 1980; J. Fletcher, 'The "Rights" to Live and to Die' in M. Kohl (ed.), *Beneficient Euthanasia*, Prometheus, Buffalo, N.Y., 1975; Richard A. McCormick, 'The Quality of Life, The Sanctity of Life', *Hastings Center Report*, February 1978; W. O. Spitzer *et al.*, *Measuring the Quality of Life of Cancer Patients — A Concise QL-Index for Use by Physicians*, Paper produced with a grant from the Commonwealth Department of Health, Canberra, undated.

20 As cited in M. O'Brien Steinfels, 'In Vitro Fertilization: "Ethically Acceptable" Research', *Hastings Center Report*, June 1978, p. 6.

21 See Peter Singer, 'Animal Liberation', *The New York Review*, New York, 1975.

22 The *Age*, (Melbourne), 26 July 1979.

23 Habermas, *Legitimation Crisis*.

Chapter 5   *The Moral Status of the Embryo*

1 B. Brody, *Abortion and the Sanctity of Life: A Philosophical View*, MIT Press, Cambridge, Mass., 1975, p. 113; M. Tooley, *The Rights and Wrongs of Abortion*, 1974, p. 75; and Mary Anne Warren in R. Hunt and J. Arras (eds), *Ethical Issues in Modern Medicine*, Mayfield Publishing Co., Palo Alto, 1977, pp. 159–78.

2 L. R. Kass, 'Making Babies Revisited', *The Public Interest*, vol. 54, 1979, pp. 32–60.

3 Edward A. Langerak, 'Abortion: Listening to the Middle', *Hastings Center Report*, vol. 9, 1979, pp. 24–8.

4 S. Siegel in *Research on the Foetus*, National Commission for the Protection of Human Subjects of Biomedical and Behavioural Research, DHEW Publications no. (OS) 76–128, 1975, pp. 7–13.

5 H. T. Engelhardt, 'The Ontology of Abortion', *Ethics*, vol. 84, 1974, p. 224.

6 J. T. Noonan (ed.), *The Morality of Abortion*, Harvard University Press, Cambridge, Mass., 1970, p. 55.

7 P. Singer, *Practical Ethics*, Cambridge University Press, Cambridge, 1979, pp. 119–24.

8 Kass, 'Making Babies Revisited', pp. 32–60.

9 L. R. Kass, 'Babies by Means of In Vitro Fertilization: Unethical Experiments on the Unborn?', *New England Journal of Medicine*, vol. 285, 1971, pp. 1174–9; L. R. Kass, 'Making Babies — The New Biology and the "Old" Morality', *The Public Interest*, vol. 26, 1972, p. 28; and P. Ramsey, 'Shall We Reproduce?', *JAMA*, vol. 220, 1972, pp. 1346–50; 1480–5.

10 J. Mahoney, 'Ethical Horizons of Human Bioethical Development', *The Month*, vol. 11, 1978, pp. 327–33.

11 R. M. Hare, 'Abortion and the Golden Rule', *Philosophy and Public Affairs*, vol. 4, 1975, pp. 205–22.

12 B. Nathanson, *Aborting America*, Doubleday, New York, 1979, pp. 218–26.

13 J. Fletcher, *The Ethics of Genetic Control: Ending Reproductive Roulette*, Doubleday, Anchor Books, New York, 1974, p. 139.

14 Singer, *Practical Ethics*, pp. 119–24.

15 P. Ramsey in J. Rachels (ed.), *Moral Problems*, Harper & Row, New York, 1975, p. 38.

16 D. Callahan, *Abortion: Law, Choice and Morality*, Macmillan Co., New York, 1970, p. 375; and P. Ramsey, 'Abortion: A Review Article', *Thomist*, vol. 37, 1973, pp. 174–226.

17 A. E. Hellegers, 'Fetal Development', *Theological Studies*, vol. 31, 1970, pp. 3–9.

18 Ramsey, 'Abortion: A Review Article', pp. 174–226.

19 Noonan (ed.), *The Morality of Abortion*, p. 55.

20 St Thomas Aquinas, *Summa Theologiae*, I, 118, art. 2, ad 2.

21 J. Donceel, 'Immediate Animation and Delayed Hominization', *Theological Studies*, vol. 31, 1970, pp. 76–105; and G. R. Dunstan, *The Artifice of Ethics*, SCM Press, London, 1974, p. 69.

22 G. Grisez, *Abortion: the Myths, the Realities and the Arguments*, Corpus Books, New York, 1972, pp. 282–306.

23 K. Rahner, *Theological Investigations IX*, Darton, Longman and Todd, London, 1975, p. 236.

24 S. Congregation for the Doctrine of the Faith, Declaration on Abortion, note 19 in O. M. Liebard (ed.), *Official Catholic Teachings: Love and Sexuality*, McGrath Publishing Co., Wilmington, 1974, p. 490.

25 Noonan (ed.), *The Morality of Abortion*, p. 55.

26 Langerak, 'Abortion: Listening to the Middle'.

27 J. T. Noonan, 'Abortion and the Catholic Church: A Summary History', *Natural Law Forum*, vol. 12, 1968, pp. 85–131.

28 H. Thielecke, *The Ethics of Sex*, trans. J. W. Dobberstein, Harper & Row, New York, 1964, pp. 226–47.

29 Kass, 'Making Babies Revisited', and L. Walters, 'Human In Vitro Fertilization: A Review of the Ethical Literature', *Hastings Center Report*, vol. 9, 1979, pp. 23–43.

30 P. Singer, *Animal Liberation*, Avon, New York, 1977, chapter 1.

Chapter 6   Informed Consent by Participants

1 O. E. Guttentag, 'Ethical Problems in Human Experimentation' in E. F. Torrey (ed.), *Ethical Issues in Medicine*, Little, Brown & Co., Boston, 1968, p. 198.

2 Nuremberg Code quoted by A. W. Burton, 'Medical Ethics and the Law', Australian Medical Association Pub. Co., 1974, p. 54.

3 Burton, 'Medical Ethics and the Law', pp. 56–7.

4 M. H. Pappworth, 'Ethical Issues in Experimental Medicine' in Donald E. Cutter (ed.), *Updating Life and Death*, Boston Beacon Press, 1969.

5 W. E. May, *Human Existence, Medicine and Ethics*, Franciscan Herald Press, Chicago, 1977, p. 21.

6 P. Ramsey, *Patient as Person*, Yale University Press, London & New Haven, 1970, p. 14.

7 P. Ramsey, 'Shall We Reproduce?' 1. The Medical Ethics of in Vitro Fertilization', *Journal of the American Medical Association*, vol. 220, 1972, p. 1347.

8 J. Fletcher, 'Ethical Aspects of Genetic Controls', in T. A. Shannon (ed.), *Bioethics*, Paulist Press, New York, 1976, p. 338.

9 Fletcher, 'Ethical Aspects of Genetic Controls', p. 336.

10 Queen Victoria Medical Centre Ethics Committee, Guidelines for clinicians and scientists involved in IVF and ET.

Chapter 7   Sexual Ethics in Relation to IVF and ET

1 R. G. Edwards, 'Fertilization of Human Eggs In Vitro: Morals, Ethics and the Law', *Quarterly Review of Biology*, vol. 49, 1974, pp. 9–11.

2 L. R. Kass, 'Babies by Means of In Vitro Fertilization: Unethical Experiments on the Unborn?', *New England Journal of Medicine*, vol. 285, 1971, p. 1177.

3 P. Ramsey, 'Shall We Reproduce?', *JAMA*, vol. 220, 1972, p. 1481.

4 R. G. Edwards and D. J. Sharpe, 'Social Values and Research in Human Embryology', *Nature*, vol. 231, 1971, p. 87; and Edwards, 'Fertilization of Human Eggs In Vitro', pp. 9–11.

5 A. Comfort, *Sex in Society*, Penguin Books, Harmondsworth, 1963, pp. 26, 15.

6 Pope Pius XII in O. E. Liebard (ed.), *Official Catholic Teachings: Love and Sexuality*, McGrath Publishing Co., Wilmington, N.C., 1951, pp. 99, 117; P. Ramsey, *Fabricated Man: The Ethics of Genetic Control*, Yale University Press, New Haven and London, 1970, p. 33; and H. Thielecke, *The Ethics of Sex*, James Clarke, London, 1964, p. 251.

7 Pope Pius XII in *Official Catholic Teachings*, pp. 99, 117.

8 Thielecke, *The Ethics of Sex*, p. 251.

9 Ramsey, *Fabricated Man*, p. 33.
10 K. Menninger, *Whatever Became of Sin?*, Hawthorn Books, New York, 1973, p. 41.
11 L. R. Kass, 'Making Babies — The New Biology and the "Old" Morality', *The Public Interest*, vol. 26, 1972, p. 49.
12 A. E. Hellegers and R. A. McCormick, 'Unanswered Questions on Test Tube Life', *America*, vol. 139, 1978, p. 77.

Chapter 8   IVF and the Human Family

1 D. Callahan, 'The Moral Career of Genetic Engineering', *Hastings Center Report*, vol. 9, no. 2, April 1979, pp. 9, 21.
2 P. Ramsey, 'Manufacturing our Offspring: Weighing the Risks', *Hastings Center Report*, vol. 8, no. 5, October 1978, pp. 7ff.
3 In D. J. O'Brien and T. A. Shannon (eds), *Renewing the Earth*, Doubleday, Image Books, New York, 1977, pp. 227f.
4 The *Age*(Melbourne), 30 April 1981, p. 12.
5 In O'Brien and Shannon (eds), *Renewing the Earth*, p. 228.
6 F. H. Marsh and D. J. Self, 'In Vitro Fertilization at the Norfolk Clinic', *Hastings Center Report*, vol. 10, no. 3, June 1980, pp. 5f.
7 The *Age* (Melbourne), 30 April 1981, p. 12.
8 The *Age* (Melbourne), 4 May 1981, p. 12.
9 The *Age* (Melbourne), 9 May 1981, p. 20.
10 S. Toulmin, 'In Vitro Fertilization: Answering the Ethical Objections', *Hastings Center Report*, vol. 8, no. 5, October 1978, pp. 9ff.
11 A. MacIntyre, 'The Wrong Questions to Ask about War', *Hastings Center Report*, vol. 10, no. 6, December 1980, p. 40.
12 Cf. P. Ramsey, *The Patient as Person*, Yale University Press, New Haven and London, pp. xi–xiii.
13 B. Mitchell, *Morality — Religious and Secular*, Oxford University Press, Clarendon, 1980, chapter 11.

Chapter 9   The Created Individual

1 P. Ramsey, *Fabricated Man: The Ethics of Genetic Control*, Yale University Press, New Haven and London, 1974, p. 106.

2 Ramsey, *Fabricated Man*, p. 39.

3 J. Fletcher, 'Ethical Aspects of Genetic Controls', *New England Journal of Medicine*, vol. 285, 1971, p. 776.

4 L. R. Kass, 'New Beginnings in Life', in M. Hamilton (ed.), *The New Genetics and Future of Man*, Eerdmans Publishing, Grand Rapids, Michigan, 1972, pp. 53–4.

5 L. Walters, 'Human In Vitro Fertilization: A Review of the Literature', *Hastings Center Report*, vol. 9, no. 4, 1979, p. 25.

6 Kass, 'New Beginnings in Life', p. 54.

7 D. Callahan, 'New Beginnings in Life. A Philosopher's Response', in Hamilton (ed.), *The New Genetics and Future of Man*, p. 101.

8 C. E. Curran, *Issues in Sexual and Medical Ethics*, University of Notre Dame Press, Notre Dame and London, 1978, p. 119.

9 K. Rahner, 'Experiment Man', *Theology Digest*, February 1968, p. 58.

10 J. Fletcher, *Humanhood*, Prometheus Books, Buffalo, 1979, pp. 16–17.

11 R. A. McCormick, *How Brave A New World?*, Doubleday, New York, 1981, p. 328.

Chapter 10 Surrogate Motherhood

1 See *Marriage Act* 1958 (Vic), s. 147; *Douglas* v. *Longano* (1981) FLC 91–024.

2 R. L. Brent and M. I. Harris (eds), *Prevention of Embryonic, Fetal, and Perinatal Disease*, DHEW Publication No. (NIH) 76–853, p. 76.

3 R. Tuchmann-Duplessis, *Drug Effects on the Fetus*, ADIS Press, New York, 1975, chapter 15.

4 Brent and Harris (eds), *Prevention of Embryonic, Fetal and Perinatal Disease*, table 1, p. 68.

5 B. M. Dickens, 'The Ectogenetic Human Being: A Problem Child of Our Time', *University of Western Ontario Law Review*, vol. 18, 1979–80, p. 259.

6 J. D. Bleich, 'Contemporary Halakhic Problems', *The Library of Jewish Law & Ethics*, no. 4, Ktav, USA, p. 108.

7 D. J. Cusine, 'Some Legal Implications of Embryo Transfer', *New Law Journal*, 28 June 1979, pp. 627–8.

8 See *Registration of Births, Deaths and Marriages Act*, 1959 (Vic.). Failure to register the birth constitutes an offence under this Act, sections 50 and 51. Other states have similar provisions.

9 For example, see *Administration and Probate Act,* 1958 (Vic.) part IV, especially section 91.

10 *Chitty on Contracts* 24th edn, Sweet & Maxwell, London, 1977, par. 960; W. S. Birks, *Parent and Child*, Legal Publications Ltd, Wellington, NZ, 1952, p. 61; *Besand* v. *Narayaniah* (1914) 30 TLR 560, 562 (PC); *Humphreys* v. *Polak* (1901) 2 KB 385, 388; *Halsbury's Laws of England*, 4th edn, vol. 1, par 610.

11 It has been suggested in some jurisdictions that a contract may be enforceable in appropriate circumstances where the contract is in the best interest of the child, for example, where the parent is not in a position to furnish proper care for the child. In *Re Shirk's Estate* 350 P 2d 1, 11 (Kansas); *Nelson* v. *Wilson* 97 SW 2d 287, 291 (Texas); In *Re Book's Estate* 147 A 668, 609 (Penns.); see also *Phillips* v. *Frederick* 58 S 2d 584, 587 (Alab.) where the fact that the promisor had had the benefit of the consideration was of prime importance; and S. Williston, *A Treatise on the Law of Contracts*, 3rd edn, New York, 1957, pp. 571–2. Note that in none of the cases cited was the plaintiff or defendant seeking to enforce a promise to hand over custody of a child. In each case, the person had already divested himself or herself of custody and was seeking to establish the legal enforceability of a promise whereby the present custodian undertook to give financial support to the child or to the former custodian (in return for which he or she would receive the pleasure associated with caring for the child).

12 In *Re Shirk's Estate* 350 P 2d 1, 11–12.

13 *The Times*, 21 June 1978. A discussion of the implications of this case can be found in Cusine, 'Some Legal Implications of Embryo Transfer'.

14 'US Judge finds Baby Contract is Legitimate', The *Age* (Melbourne), 27 April 1981, p. 6.

15 'What Price Motherhood?', The *Age* (Melbourne, 4 May 1981.

16 See A. R. Holder, *Legal Issues in Pediatrics and Adolescent Medicine*, J. Wiley & Sons, USA, 1977, p. 9.

17 Dickens, 'The Ectogenetic Human Being', pp. 257–8.

18 L. R. Kass, 'Making Babies — The New Biology and the "Old" Morality', *The Public Interest*, no. 26 (Winter), 1972, p. 36; L.

Walters, 'Human In Vitro Fertilization: A Review of the Ethical Literature', *Hastings Center Report*, vol. 9, no. 4, August 1979, p. 33; and Dickens, 'The Ectogenetic Human Being', p. 258.

19 Only twenty babies were made available for adoption in 1980 at the Queen Victoria Medical Centre. In 1978 and 1979, the figure was eighteen for each year.

20 P. Reilly, 'In Vitro Fertilisation — A Legal Perspective', in A. Milunsky and G. Annas (eds), *Genetics and the Law*, Plenum Press, New York, 1976, p. 370; see contrary view of M. Revillard, 'Legal Aspects of Artificial Insemination and Embryo Transfer in French Domesic and Private International Law', in *Law and Ethics of AID and Embryo Transfer*, CIBA Foundation Symposium 17, Association of Scientific Publishers, Amsterdam, 1973, p. 87.

21 Dickens, 'The Ectogenetic Human Being', p. 261; Reilly, 'In Vitro Fertilization', p. 371.

22 A medical practitioner who carries out a medical procedure on a patient without his or her consent is guilty of the civil wrong of battery (*Reibl* v. *Hughes* (1977) 16 OR (2d) 306). To force the practitioner into breach of the law by compelling the patient to undergo treatment would be against public policy and therefore untenable.

23 On trauma associated with unintended discovery, see Day in Tony Hall (ed.), *Access to Birth Records*, ABAFA, London, 1980, pp. 22–3.

24 Day in *Access*, p. 32, esp. parts 10, 12 and 20; *Adoption Legislation Review Committee (Vic.)* Working Party, part 1, December 1980, pp. 62–89, par. 5; C. Picton and M. Bieske-Voss, Person in Question: Adoptees in Search of Origins, Unpublished, Monash University, 1980, 11.1 and 11.2.

Chapter 11   Cloning, Ectogenesis, and Hybrids

1 D. Rorvik, quoted by R. G. McKinnell, *Cloning: A Biologist Reports*, University of Minnesota Press, Minneapolis, 1979, p. 5.

2 J. B. Gurdon, 'Transplanted Nuclei and Cell Differentiation', *Scientific American*, vol. 219, 1968, pp. 24–35.

3 L. E. Karp, *Genetic Engineering: Threat or Promise*, Nelson-Hall, Chicago, 1976, pp. 161–206.

4 Ibid.

5 D. M. Mackay, *Human Science and Human Dignity*, Hodder and Stoughton, London, 1979, p. 69.

6 P. Ramsey, *Fabricated Man: The Ethics of Genetic Control*, Yale University Press, New Haven and London, 1975, p. 89.

7 F. Rosner, 'Recombinant DNA, Cloning, Genetic Engineering and Judaism', *New York State Journal of Medicine*, vol. 79, 1979, pp. 1439–44.

8 Ramsey, *Fabricated Man*, p. 89; and B. Häring, *Manipulation: Ethical Boundaries of Medical, Behavioural and Genetic Manipulation*, St Paul Publications, England, 1975, pp. 203–6.

9 Rosner, 'Recombinant DNA', pp. 1439–44.

10 J. Lederberg, 'Biological Innovation and Genetic Intervention', in J. A. Behnke (ed.), *Challenging Biomedical Problems: Directions Towards their Solution*, Oxford University Press, New York, 1972, p. 23.

11 J. Fletcher, *The Ethics of Genetic Control: Ending Reproductive Roulette*, Doubleday, Anchor Books, New York, 1974, pp. 147–87.

12 R. G. McKinnell, *Cloning: A Biologist Reports*, University of Minnesota Press, Minneapolis, 1979, pp. 50–77.

13 W. Ironside and D. Mushin, Determinants of Interactive Disturbance between Mothers and their Premature Babies (in press).

14 Karp, *Genetic Engineering*, pp. 161–206.

15 S. Firestone, *The Dialectic of Sex: The Case for Feminist Revolution*, Bantam Books, New York, 1971, pp. 196–200.

16 R. G. Edwards, 'Fertilization of Human Eggs In Vitro: Morals, Ethics and the Law', *Quarterly Review of Biology*, vol. 49, 1974, pp. 3–14.

17 G. Leach, *The Biocrats: Implications of Medical Progress*, Penguin Books, Harmondsworth, 1972, p. 116.

18 Fletcher, *The Ethics of Genetic Control*, pp. 147–87.

19 L. Walters, 'Human In Vitro Fertilization: A Review of the Ethical Literature', *Hastings Center Report*, August 1979, pp. 23–43.

Glossary

abortion
Spontaneous or induced termination of pregnancy before the foetus is capable of survival outside the womb.

AID (artificial insemination donor)
The injection of seminal fluid, obtained from a donor by masturbation, into the upper vagina, canal of the neck of the womb or into the cavity of the womb itself. In this case, the man producing the semen specimen is *not* the husband of the woman being inseminated and is usually anonymous as far as she is concerned. This method is mainly used to aid conception when the husband is infertile or when he has or carries a genetic disorder which has a high risk of being transmitted to his children.

AIH (artificial insemination husband)
The injection of seminal fluid, obtained from the husband by masturbation, into the upper vagina, canal of the neck of the womb or into the cavity of the womb itself. This method is mainly used to aid conception when the husband cannot achieve or maintain erection of the penis rendering normal intercourse impossible.

amniocentesis
The passage of a needle into the cavity of the womb and withdrawal of 10-20 ml of amniotic fluid from around the developing foetus at 15-16 weeks of pregnancy. The procedure is used to diagnose some abnormalities of the foetus at an early stage of pregnancy, by analysis of the contents of the fluid.

a priori
Reasoning from that which is prior, either as a condition of thought or as a condition of existence —— logically or chronologically.

blastocyst
The early embryo at the stage when it consists of a ball of cells containing a cavity filled with fluid. This stage occurs about five days after fertilization when the embryo is ready to embed in the lining of the womb.

covenant
A mutual agreement, often in writing.

clone
A colony of cells identical with and arising from a single parent cell. Cloning is an asexual method of reproduction which is not yet possible in higher species of animals or man.

congenital
Used to describe something with which one is born; usually a deformity or disease.

cognitive
Pertaining to that activity of the mind that 'knows' things; an awareness of the processes of thinking and perceiving including understanding and reasoning.

comatose
Affected with coma; a state of complete loss of consciousness from which the affected person cannot be roused by any ordinary external stimulus.

chromosomes
Thread-like structures in the cell nucleus that carry the genetic information of the cell in a linear array of functional units, called genes. The chromosomes are complexes of proteins and are not visible under the microscope as separate entities until the cell commences division, when they appear as rod-like structures.

conceptus
The developing product of conception throughout pregnancy.

custody
The guarding or caring of a child.

demographic
Pertaining to study of populations.

DNA
The abbreviation for de-oxy-ribonucleic acid, the hereditary protein material of the cell found in the chromosomes of the cell nucleus.

deontological
Pertaining to the theory of duty or obligation which is not entirely dependent on the theory of value, e.g. the theory that an action may be known to be right without a consideration of the goodness of its consequences.

Down's syndrome
A chromosomal disorder resulting in mental retardation and various physical defects.

ectogenesis
Growth of the foetus outside of the human body, without the need for the maternal womb at any stage.

egg
The female cell arising in the ovary, which when fertilized by a male sperm cell, results in an embryo.

egg follicle
The egg follicle is a small fluid-filled cyst that houses the egg cell, in the ovary. It ruptures at the time of ovulation to allow escape of the egg.

embryo
The early developing fertilized egg that is growing into another individual of the species. In man the term ''embryo'' is usually restricted to the period of development from fertilization until the end of the eighth week of pregnancy.

embryo transfer (ET)
The transfer of the early embryo, after fertilization of the egg in vitro in the laboratory, to the womb. This is usually done at the two to four cell stage of embryonic development about 24-36 hours after fertilization.

empirical
Relating to experience; having reference to actual facts.

ethics
The study of the nature of values, rights and obligations.

ex corpo
Out of the body.

ex nuptial
Out of marriage.

extracorporeal gestation
Growth of the embryo and foetus without relation to the body.

extrauterine
Without relation to the uterus or womb.

fallopian tube
The uterine tube that conveys the egg, fertilized or unfertilized, from the ovary to the womb. Gabriele Fallopio was an anatomist who was born in Padua, Italy, in 1523.

fecundity
Fruitfulness.

foetus
The term applied to the embryo from the end of the eighth week of pregnancy up to birth.

gamete
A cell concerned with reproduction e.g. the egg and sperm cells.

gene
One of a series of protein units arranged in linear order on the chromosomes of the cell nucleus. Genes are self-reproducible at cell division and are thought to be the ultimate determinants of the characteristics of the organism.

genetic
Pertaining to the gene or genes.

genetic engineering
The manipulation of genes by scientific means in the laboratory.

genotype
The genetic constitution.

genus
A group of closely related species or a single species of plant or animal life.

high risk pregnancy
A pregnancy at risk of being lost as a result of maternal or foetal disease.

homo sapiens
Human species.

hubris
Arrogance arising from pride and often involving insolence.

hybrid
The individual resulting from the union of two different species.

infertility
The inability to conceive and sometimes, in the case of the woman, to bear children.

in vivo
In the living situation.

in vitro fertilization (IVF)
Fertilization outside the human body in the laboratory.

intra-uterine device (IUD)
A mechanical device placed in the cavity of the womb to prevent pregnancy.

ipso facto
By that very fact.

Kantianism
The philosophy of Immanuel Kant (1724-1804), often referred to as the 'critical' philosophy —— that which seeks to find out what it is possible for any mind like the human mind to know. In ethics, Kant emphasised the role of reason and said that moral laws were based on a 'categorical imperative that applies to all rational beings'.

laparoscopy
The operation whereby a telescope is passed into the carbon-dioxide gas-filled abdominal and pelvic cavities under general or local anaesthesia. This enables inspection of the internal organs and the collection of human eggs from the ovaries.

Lesch-Nyhan disease
A hereditary disease due to deficiency of a protein and characterised by mental retardation, self-mutilation and nervous system abnormalities.

liability
The state of being subject to an obligation.

masturbation
Stimulation of the sexual organs to produce orgasm.

menopause
The cessation of the monthly blood loss from the womb.

menstrual cycle
The cycle of events occurring regularly at monthly intervals in the human female genital organs and characterised most readily by the periodic disintegration of the lining of the womb resulting in blood loss from the vagina once every 28 days or thereabouts.

miscarriage
The spontaneous loss of an early pregnancy at any stage before the twentieth week after conception.

moral
Relating to character or conduct that is considered to be good or evil.

nucleus
The structure in the cell that governs cell function.

ontology
The study of 'being' or of what exists; the science of the essence of things.

ovary
One or two such organs bearing the egg cells and situated within the pelvic cavity.

parthenogenesis
Non-sexual reproduction by means of an egg independent of fertilization by the male.

placenta
The organ housed within the womb during pregnancy through which the developing foetus carries on its vital functions; often referred to as the 'afterbirth' because it is delivered soon after the birth of the baby.

pragmatics
An approach which judges things in terms of their usefulness for other purposes.

primate
A member of one of the species of the highest order of mammals, including lemurs, monkeys, anthropoid apes and man.

procreation
The production of offspring.

progeny
Offspring.

pronuclei
The nucleus of the mature egg and the nucleus of the sperm head after it has penetrated the egg cell at the time of fertilization are called pronuclei: after they fuse, the single nucleus in the egg is then termed the cleavage nucleus.

puberty
The stage in a person's life during which the sex glands (testicles or ovaries) become active.

sanctity
The quality of being sacred or holy and hence inviolable.

semen
The fluid carrying sperm.

sexual roulette
Refers to the random nature of normal human reproduction in contrast to selective breeding for certain characteristics.

situation ethics
The ethical approach to a problem determined by the circumstances at the time rather than by *a priori* considerations or divine laws.

speciesist
A person biased towards a being simply because it is a member of his or her own species.

sperm
The male cells of reproduction.

surrogate mother
A substitute mother who has agreed to bear a child for another woman who cannot bear children herself.

utilitarianism
The view that the right act is the act that will actually or probably produce the greatest amount of pleasure or happiness in the world at large.

uterus
Womb.

zygote
The early stage of the embryo after fertilization.

Contributors

Mrs Isabel Bainbridge is a patient in the IVF programme.

Rev. B. E. Carey, BA, BD, is a Uniting Church Minister within the Ivanhoe Parish, Melbourne.

Rev. Fr W. J. Daniel, SJ, MA, STD, is Principal of the Jesuit Theological College and Lecturer in the United Faculty of Theology, Melbourne.

Rev. Dr J. A. Henley, BA, BD, PhD, is Dean of the Melbourne College of Divinity.

Rev. Dr B. Johnstone, PhD, is Lecturer in Moral Theology at the Yarra Theological Union, Melbourne, and Visiting Associate Professor at the Catholic University of America, Washington.

Ms Helga Kuhse, BA (Hons), is a Research Fellow in the Centre for Human Bioethics, Monash University.

Professor J. F. Leeton, MBBS, DCH, FCRS, FRACS, FRCOG, MGO, FRACOG, is Associate Professor in the Department of Obstetrics and Gynaecology, Monash University.

Rev. Dr J. L. Morgan, BA (Hons), DipEd (Melb.), MA, DPhil (Oxon), is Ecumenical Chaplain to the University of Melbourne, Senior Tutor at St Hilda's College, and Lecturer in the United Faculty of Theology, Melbourne.

Alan A. Rassaby, BA, LLB, is a Research Fellow in the Centre for Human Bioethics, Monash University.

Peter Roberts is the science reporter of the *Age* newspaper, Melbourne.

Professor Peter Singer is Chairman, Department of Philosophy, Monash University.

Dr A. O. Trounson, MSc (NSW), PhD (Syd.), is a Lecturer in the Department of Obstetrics and Gynaecology, Monash University.

Professor W. A. W. Walters, MBBS, PhD, FROG, FRACOG, is Associate Professor in the Department of Obstetrics and Gynaecology, Monash University.

Professor Carl Wood, MBBS, FRCS, FROG, FRACOG, Chairman, Department of Obstetrics and Gynaecology, Monash University.